Judgment 3

21/8/03

Caring for the dying
MICHAEL BARBATO

With gratitude and love
to Ann, Claire, Ruth, James, Moira and David

Caring for the dying
MICHAEL BARBATO

MCGRAW HILL BOOK COMPANY Sydney
New York San Francisco Auckland Bogotá Caracas
Lisbon London Madrid Mexico City Milan Montreal
New Delhi San Juan Singapore Tokyo Toronto

McGraw·Hill Australia

A Division of The McGraw·Hill Companies

Text © 2002 Michael Barbato
Illustrations and Design © 2002 McGraw-Hill Australia Pty Limited
Additional owners of copyright material are credited on the Acknowledgments page.

National Library of Australia Cataloguing-in-Publication data:

Barbato, Michael
Caring for the Dying

Includes index.
ISBN 0 074 71214 4.

1. Terminal care. 2. Terminally ill. 3. Death – Psychological aspects.
I. Title.

362.175

Published in Australia by
McGraw-Hill Australia Pty Limited
4 Barcoo Street, Roseville NSW 2069, Australia
Publishing Manager: Meiling Voon
Production Editor: Rosemary McDonald
Editor: Jo Rudd
Proofreader: Tim Learner
Indexer: Diane Harriman
Design (interior and cover): Jenny Pace
Cover image: Getty Images Pty Ltd
Typeset in Goudy by Jenny Pace
Printed on 80 gsm woodfree by Pantech Limited, Hong Kong.

Contents

Acknowledgments

*t*his book was once nothing more than an ambitious thought. I am grateful to the many people who have helped make it a reality. I particularly wish to thank Ann for her support and inspiration, Claire for her unstinting faith and helpful comments and to Ruth, James and David for their continued interest and suggestions. I would also like to express my gratitude to Meiling Voon and Rosemary McDonald of McGraw Hill Pty Limited for their hard work, patience and understanding and the professional and sensitive manner they guided me throughout the whole process. Finally a sincere thanks to those I have cared for, for allowing me to be present at such a crucial time of their life.

CREDIT Michael Leunig extracts from the *Common Prayer Collection* by Michael Leunig, HarperCollins Publishers

God bless this tiny little boat
And me who travels in it.
It stays afloat for years and years
And sinks within a minute.

And so the soul in which we sail,
Unknown by years of thinking,
Is deeply felt and understood
The minute that it's sinking.

MICHAEL LEUNIG, COMMON PRAYER COLLECTION

How shall I know the way of all things?
By what is inside me.

LAO TZU

Prologue

*a*s a palliative care doctor I am often asked by patients and their relatives how I can do this type of work. There are times when I wonder too, particularly as many people, doctors and nurses included, are so uncomfortable with death. I suspect the answer lies in the journey my life has taken.

I have clear memories as a young child of accompanying my parents to the homes of their mothers as each was dying, one of stomach cancer, the other of heart disease. I watched them tend my grandmothers and then assist with the ritual washing and dressing after death. I was barely old enough to understand the significance of the occasion but it was clear even then that people we love die. I was overwhelmed to see my parents crying but what struck me most was the amount of love and support such a sad event could generate. The rituals and customs my Italian parents and relatives immersed themselves in suggested that death was no stranger. Although unwelcome, it was treated as a part of life and given due respect.

In the following years my family had several uncomfortable brushes with death. My twin sister was run over by a car but miraculously survived unscathed. My eldest brother was involved in a motor vehicle accident in which another person was killed, another brother survived a life-threatening bout of encephalitis and I nearly drowned while swimming in a lake. This was a difficult time for my parents.

At that time it seemed as if our family had cheated death. I believed death had no power over us and, as a young boy, I challenged it to show its face! My bravado seemed to work and death took a break.

It revisited several years later when one of my secondary

school classmates failed to show at school, another's sister died of leukaemia and another drowned while trying to save children in his charge. These sudden and unexpected deaths were unsettling, but the news that another friend had killed his mother made it all incomprehensible. Death revealed a tragic side that I had not appreciated. Death was not simply a mysterious void that claimed the aged, but was ever present and could not be denied. I now feared death and began to exercise caution in what I did.

After graduation in 1966 I began work in a large Sydney hospital where death was an everyday occurrence. At first I found this overwhelming and emotionally draining but gradually I learnt not to get involved and became immune to its presence and its effects. This helped me to survive but led to a form of clinical detachment that facilitated objectivity but undermined my ability to see beyond the patient.

This approach was severely tested over ensuing years as five close colleagues died suddenly and at an early age as a result of illness, accident or suicide. Closer to home one of my relatives made two unsuccessful attempts to end their life – on both occasions I found him and initiated resuscitation.

Death had really made its presence known. For the first time I began to wonder about the meaning of life and the significance of death. I also questioned the work I was doing and what contribution I was making to the care of people.

Intent on using my recently acquired specialist skills, I moved to a large country town with my young family in tow. In no time I was busier than I needed to be and only now realise it was because I needed my patients more than they needed me. My sense of self depended on being busy and on what others thought of me. Death was still always present but now I saw it as the enemy, an enemy I mistakenly believed could be defeated. I saved many lives but others died. My response was simply to try harder.

About this time a young man was admitted to my unit. He'd had a heart attack but, as his condition seemed stable, I reassured him and his wife and young family that all would be well. How wrong I was. Over the next week this man's heart stopped many times. Each time he was brought back to life. I continued to assure him that he would be all right, knowing deep down that this could be false hope. I took it upon myself not to tell them of the danger signs or the distinct possibility of death, even though his and his wife's anxiety was palpable.

The man died. My first thought was that I'd failed him medically, even though all my decisions had been guided by specialists from Sydney. It was only when his wife and children were saying farewell to their dead husband and father that I realised I had not failed medically but had allowed my fears and ambitions to cloud my judgment and care. By giving false hope I had deprived them of the chance to say goodbye and prepare for the inevitable. I had abused their trust and failed them in their time of greatest need. I may have become an expert in the care of the body but I had been oblivious and insensitive to the needs of mind, heart and soul.

Several years of anguish followed when I reached deep within to find some meaning to my life and a reason to continue the work that occupied a large part of it. A change of town and a new job did not provide the answers and only exacerbated the problems I'd hoped to leave behind.

It was at this time that our fourth child, Moira, died unexpectedly of SIDS (cot death) at the age of one month. The effect this had on us all cannot be described. Moira's death was as incomprehensible as it was tragic, and a large part of us died with her. My wife, Ann, our children and I struggled to come to terms with her death. For my part, several work changes and two bouts of depression only served to remind me of the despair that had descended on us. The sudden death of Ann's mother, the protracted death of her father from cancer as we cared for him at home, my father's death and the death of several friends rocked our lives even more. Ann and I realised we had to make changes to our life and that I could not continue with the work I was doing.

In 1989, fourteen years after Moira's death, we left our beloved country town and many dear friends and headed for Sydney. This radical and paradoxical change was so that I could start work as a palliative care doctor. I thought I had seen enough death to last a lifetime, but I seemed incomprehensibly drawn to it.

The thirteen years I have since spent in palliative care have presented me with some of the most rewarding and challenging times in my life. Working in palliative care has stretched me to the limit, but being with people as they confront their death is a privilege few have. In some strange and mysterious way they have helped me rediscover a part of myself that was for some time lost. This book is a tribute to all those people.

Books that deal with death and dying have little to recommend them. They rarely make the bestseller list. So why write another book on a subject most consider morbid? How can it benefit you as you care for your sick relative or friend?

What dying people fear most is the loneliness that may accompany their dying. The inability to share their fears, anxieties and wishes and to be blatantly honest about their life and death is often more painful than the thought of death itself.

After reading this book, I hope that those of you who care for a dying person will be more aware and able to 'hear' what is in their heart and mind, and less afraid to talk about death. After almost forty years of caring for the sick and dying the one thing I have learnt is their need for authentic human contact. Dying is hard, but to die with all one's thoughts and emotions locked inside is tragic.

I would like to thank all those I have cared for and their families. Allowing me to enter into their life at such a vulnerable time has helped me to see the value of trust, love and a life fully lived. I also wish to thank Ann, my partner in life, for being 'nothing less than thee' and our children whose individual beauty has given us countless joys and endless rewards. Family, colleagues and friends have sustained me in many ways and I give thanks that they too have been part of my journey.

1 Introduction

> Science says we must live and seeks the means of prolonging, increasing, facilitating and amplifying life, of making it tolerable and acceptable. Wisdom says we must die and seeks how to make us die well.
>
> MIGUEL DE UNAMUNO

Tom was in his mid-sixties and had retired from work less than one year before. He was admitted to the palliative care ward because of breathing difficulties from lung cancer, diagnosed several months earlier. The cancer had not responded to chemotherapy and radiotherapy, and when Tom arrived he was thin and gaunt and looked most unwell. I was not surprised when he told me he had come into the ward to die. Such candour is not rare among those confronted with the prospect of dying but what did intrigue me was his refusal to have any treatment to ease his breathlessness. With my medical hat firmly in place I explained how morphine and other treatments could help his breathing and make dying that little bit easier. He looked at me, just as my father did when I had missed the point he was trying to make. Between breaths, he declared with steely resolve, 'I have heard so much about this dying business, I want to see what it is all about. I want to be awake when it happens and I want to do it well.'

*a*t the time I was surprised by Tom's comment, particularly his request to remain awake. I thought this was unusual. His desire to die well was not so. This desire is as old as civilisation, shown by the many treatises devoted to the problems of death and dying. The oldest of these, the Egyptian, Tibetan and Maya Books of the Dead date back 5000, 1200 and 1100 years respectively. The western equivalent, *Ars Moriendi* (*The Art of Dying*), was popular throughout Europe in the fifteenth century and, as with the more ancient texts, emphasised the need to prepare for death.

Given the improvements in medical care, the chances of dying well should be much better now than 500 or even 50 years ago. But that does not seem to be the case. According to Daniel Callahan, 'Death is now harder to predict, more difficult to manage, the source of more and more moral dilemmas and nasty choices, and spiritually more productive of anguish, ambivalence and uncertainty'. Dying may be less painful but the prospect of dying well today remains more of a hope than an expectation. Woody Allen spoke humorously but revealingly when he said, 'It's not that I am afraid of death, I just do not want to be there when it happens.' This desire to hide from the reality of death is universal and says as much about our unwillingness to forgo life as it does about a fear of the unknown. We fear only that which we do not know and for most of us death is certainly more of a stranger now than it was at any time in the past.

Tom's wish to die well was not that his death should be 'painless' but that it should be consistent with his wishes and in keeping with his way of life. Like each of us, Tom had, in his own special way, made his mark on life and in the face of death he wanted this to be recognised and respected. A death free of pain and suffering was no doubt important but not at the expense of dignity and integrity. The values Tom lived by were the same values he wanted upheld while dying. To do this he needed understanding, and in part his request to die well was that he not be coerced or compromised at this time of greatest need.

Such courage is not unusual but is rarely found in those who do not accept the inevitability of death. Acceptance or resignation is the first and most essential step in dying well.

Many of us live in fear of death or deny its very existence; ironically, it is this failure to integrate it into our life that can make dying such a frightening and overwhelming experience. The paradox is that children and adults see more deaths in one year's TV viewing than any doctor sees in a lifetime of medical practice but, despite or because of this, death has become a matter of fiction rather than fact, something that only happens to others.

The only thing we can be certain of at birth is that one day we shall die. Rather than deny death, we can instead see it as a beacon that guides and helps us to become more attuned to the fullness and beauty of life. Death brings life into focus and gives it meaning. It is the fulfilment of a life, not merely its culmination. Preparing for death does not draw the curtains on life but opens them wide, inviting us to appreciate and engage life, to live more intensely and be fully aware of all that surrounds us.

This book is written to honour those such as Tom who show great courage in the face of death and remain determined not to be defeated by something we all fear yet rarely prepare for. Tom's determination to do it well, even though fear may have been overwhelming, is unusual and has led me to believe that dying may be easier if people were better prepared for what lay ahead. I wonder why the art of dying well is such a neglected topic. Have you ever thought about what it would be like to die and why death is given so little attention when it is clearly of major importance to all? Fear rather than irrelevancy is what sets the agenda, even when our own death awaits us. The head-in-the-sand approach espoused by Woody Allen does not overcome fear of death; ultimately, it will have to be confronted before dying well is possible.

Nathan was an imposing figure prior to his surgery for bowel cancer. In his youth Nathan had defied and possibly denied the existence of death as he took to his motorcycle and 'burnt up' many a stretch in the western suburbs of Sydney. He had lost a leg in the process but remained defiant and undefeated until the cancer that had taken over his body started to take over his life. Nathan was frightened but it was hard for a man who had previously feared no person or thing to admit this. Instead, he withdrew to his bedroom or garage but also into himself and it was there, I suspect, he fought his battles. As he edged closer to death the fear was almost palpable and it was clear he wanted to talk but never did. Maybe he did not have the words to tell any of us exactly how he felt. Then, during one of my routine visits, Nathan asked if he was doing it right. I could almost feel the relief in his voice. While he couldn't talk about death, he could talk about it as a job that he needed to complete and, like Tom, he wanted to do it well. It might have parallels with the first time he sat on a motorbike—could he handle it? In his earlier years he may have been too proud and macho to ask for help, but not now. In his own way, he was asking for help so he could overcome fear and die well. And he did die well, with a level of courage that exceeded anything he could have believed possible. I had the impression that so much of Nathan's courage was directed to confronting fear that only when he openly acknowledged his need for help could he direct his courage to dying well.

Death resembles birth in so many ways. Both are processes defined and controlled by nature, and accompanied by fear and anticipation. Each journey is different, of varying duration and ends in a transition, one into life and the other into death. While the birth journey is well understood and divided into known stages, the death journey is less clearly defined but nonetheless has its own stages of labour. In western society, many birth and death journeys are made within a hospital but, increasingly, there is a move away from this clinical environment into the home.

Whatever the setting, every journey is made alone but is assisted and sometimes made possible by the actions of an intermediary. It is at this point that the similarity starts to fade.

Birthing classes prepare mothers for what lies ahead and highly skilled midwives ensure, as far as possible, a safe natural birth. But there are no dying classes and few people, even doctors, are skilled in the art of facilitating a safe and natural death. This was not always the case; in years past parents and extended family not only acted as midwives at birth but frequently delivered their dying child or other family member into death. This is still so in many poorer countries but, in Australia and other so-called developed countries, men and women in white coats preside over the death of those we love as we sit by helpless, watching something we do not fully understand.

 Birth and death are the bookends of life.

M COLLETT, *At Home with Dying*

As with Tom, dying may proceed naturally, needing little in the way of outside interference. That, however, is the exception rather than the rule with assistance often necessary for physical, psychological or spiritual 'complications'. While much of this help comes from a professional source, its implementation frequently falls to the carer who, in essence, acts as the midwife. This midwife, unlike her birthing counterpart, is inexperienced but will be called upon to make decisions and carry out treatments that are unfamiliar and onerous. The aim of this book is to give carers greater insight into the wider dimensions of the dying process and help each one become the skilled midwife in the death of their loved one.

This book addresses many of the questions put to me as a palliative care physician. Concerns almost invariably relate to physical care and how it can best be delivered under changing and challenging circumstances. Much of the material thus relates to physical comfort but, as this is inextricably linked to emotional and spiritual issues, a more holistic approach is taken on most matters. I have written particularly but not exclusively for those caring for someone with cancer but, as the most important issues around dying centre on a person's humanity rather than their illness, I hope the book will benefit all carers irrespective of their loved one's diagnosis. Whatever your reasons for picking up this book, I hope you find something of value from which you can draw strength and a measure of reassurance while continuing that most privileged of all tasks—journeying with a fellow human being as they die.

I am not a counsellor, a psychologist or an expert on the subject of death. I have experienced loss in my immediate family and have had the privilege of caring for many people who have died, as well as supporting their family and friends throughout the process. In writing this book I have drawn on this experience, not necessarily to give answers to problems but to provide information that may empower you in your task.

This book is not meant to glamorise death. Loss of life comes at an unimaginable and immeasurable cost. Pain and grief are inescapable and the strength required to see the process through to its completion is as great for family and friends as for the dying person. Grahame Jones, in his book *Magnanimous Despair*, says, 'The strength I need to die is nothing compared to that which will be required of those who must go on living.' And so it is. Death spells the end of pain for the one that dies but heralds a new and surreal form of living for those left behind. Death is a momentous time in any person's life. Bearing this in mind, the book discusses some of the ways your loved one's dying may affect you and how you can care for yourself as you continue this most loving but difficult of all tasks.

Recognising that we care for people, not patients, I have tried to avoid the use of the impersonal 'patient'. At times it was unavoidable and I apologise for when the personal was sacrificed for the sake of clarity. The terms 'palliative care unit' and 'hospice' are used interchangeably throughout the book. All case reports are true but the names, other than

Steve's, have been changed to try to ensure anonymity. Steve asked that his name be retained if ever I wrote about him.

 The strong are here to look after the weak and the weak here to teach the strong.

TIM WINTON, *Cloudstreet*

2 Palliative care

At the heart of modern medicine is a conflict about the place and meaning of death in human life.

DANIEL CALLAHAN

*O*nce the natural and expected consequence of illness, death is now often the unnatural end of a series of treatments that, if not intended to cure, seek at least to prolong life. This is especially true with cancer where people may go from one form of treatment to another, hoping beyond hope that a cure will ultimately be found. When medicine has nothing further to offer, fear accompanies disappointment and an uncertain future casts a shadow over the life of those affected. In this setting, modern medicine seems to have lost its way as it struggles to reconcile the value of human life with the place and meaning of death. Does it continue to offer successive treatments even when the potential for improvement diminishes and toxicity increases, or does it accept Daniel Callahan's ideal that preservation of life at any cost does not outweigh the value of a peaceful death?

Until quite recently those who were dying of a chronic illness were anomalies in a health system that is singularly orientated towards cure. It seems that medicine has little if anything to offer when cure is no longer the ideal, and those who 'fail to respond' often become casualties of a model that overlooks the need for care. Medicine has conquered many diseases but it has lost track of the indisputable fact that it will never conquer death and that a peaceful death is as important as the pursuit of cure. Dr Elisabeth Kübler-Ross and Dame Cicely Saunders had long recognised the importance of a peaceful death and in 1967 Dame Cicely Saunders created a model of care that sought to address the numerous unmet needs of those who were dying. This model of care is now known as palliative care or the modern hospice movement.

The palliative care model has grown and spread worldwide but, just as medicine has changed, so too has palliative care. In its formative years, people dying of cancer were almost the sole beneficiaries of this form of care. The model we have today is more inclusive and offers care to those with diseases other than cancer, people whose disease is not terminal and to whom quality of life is as important as length of life. These changes have not only resulted in better and more holistic care of those with an 'incurable' illness but has slowly awakened health care professions and society to the inevitability of death and the importance of caring for those who are dying.

Palliative care has been an integral part of the Australian health care system for more than thirty years and services now exist in all capital and most regional centres. Despite this, confusion still exists in the mind of the public and also within the health care profession as to what palliative care is, what it does and how it interfaces with current services, particularly the patient's own general practitioner (GP). Care of the dying is complex and challenging enough without the added confusion of deciding who you can call upon in time of need. Those new to the caring role will have had little exposure to palliative care and the following information is offered to maximise your ability to care for the one you love. Palliative care cannot prevent death but does, as Callahan says, 'Change the way people are cared for at the end of life and substantially reduces the burden of illness'.

WHAT IS PALLIATIVE CARE?
*Palliative care is a philosophy as much as a practice. It sets out to
improve the quality of life of those with a life-threatening illness.
The core values as set out by Palliative Care Australia are as
follows:*

*Palliative care is the active total care of people whose disease is
not responsive to active treatment. Care is delivered by
coordinated medical, nursing and allied health services that are
provided, where possible, in the environment of the person's
choice. Control of pain, of other symptoms and of psychological,
social, emotional and spiritual problems is paramount.*

*The goal of palliative care is achievement of the best possible
quality of life for patients and their families and friends. Many
aspects of palliative care are also applicable earlier in the course
of the illness in conjunction with treatment aimed at cure.*

Who provides palliative care?

A large number of people provide palliative care, but the most
important by far is you, the carer. Relatives, friends, the GP
and the community nurses are also vital members of this team
and are the ones most likely to be called upon in times of
need. GPs are ideally placed to do much of the medical work
as they have the appropriate medical knowledge and are in
regular contact with other specialists. They are likely to know
the family and be familiar with some of the intimate factors
and dynamics that underlie the social, emotional and
existential grief. Nurses are available to help with the physical
care, monitor day-to-day progress and assess your loved one's
response to treatment. They can answer your questions and
liaise with the GP or other members of the palliative care
team. Relatives and friends offer physical and moral support
and can be there when times are tough.

You may be surprised to find that you, the carer, feature so
high in the list of providers but, in the home situation, you
oversee all the care and deliver much of it yourself. You not

only fulfil a vital role in ensuring that pain and other symptoms are controlled, but you are also the main source of emotional comfort and, from my experience, the person most sought after in times of crisis.

Other members of the team include specialist palliative care nurses and doctors, social workers, counsellors, physiotherapist, occupational therapist, pastoral care workers and volunteers. All these people are available to help with complicated problems, supply equipment (such as hospital beds, commodes) or provide essential back up for the GP. Referral to a palliative care team carries with it a referral to all team members. The referral is usually made by the GP but in urgent or unusual circumstances referral will be accepted from a carer or relative. Contact details for your nearest palliative care service can be obtained from your GP or from your state or territory association (see Appendix).

A special mention must be made of the enormous contribution volunteers make to palliative care and how they can assist you. Volunteers come from every walk of life and bring with them their own life skills and experiences. Many of them have been in a similar position to you and are therefore well attuned to the difficulties of being a carer. Every volunteer participates in a special training program that prepares them for the emotional and physical challenges they may encounter and explains their clearly defined roles and responsibilities. They can be of enormous assistance. To find out more, contact your nearest palliative care service and ask to speak to the volunteer coordinator. He or she will tell you about the service and what it can offer.

Here are a few of the ways volunteers can assist you at home.

◆ *Daytime respite.* This provides you with the opportunity to shop, visit friends or pamper yourself at leisure, knowing a responsible and skilled person is with your loved one, giving the necessary companionship and care. This respite usually takes place in your home but is also available through specialised palliative care day centres, if one exists in your area. The latter occasionally offer transport to and from the centre if it is required.

◆ *Night respite*. If you have had a few rough nights and are short of sleep, some but not all volunteer services offer night respite. A volunteer stays overnight and deals with any problem that may arise while you catch up on sleep.

◆ *Companionship* for you and your loved one, particularly if you are socially or geographically isolated.

◆ *Provide transport* to and from appointments if no other means of travel is available or practical.

Is palliative care only for those close to death?

In its early years palliative care was almost exclusively concerned with the care of those who were close to death. Most were treated within hospices and very few returned home. Palliative care was therefore seen as terminal care and referral carried with it the understanding that death was near. In keeping with this, people were accepted for palliative care only if they had a life expectancy of less than three months.

Those days have long passed and referral to palliative care no longer depends on when death may occur or, more correctly, when the doctor thinks death will occur. Contemporary palliative care focuses on quality of life and symptom control, and this can be as important in the earlier stages of life-threatening disease as it is around the time of death. That is not to say the care of people at the end of life is given a lesser status. The importance of a good death is still an integral part of palliative care but it is now part of a continuum of care and assumes increasing importance as a person's health deteriorates. It is not palliative care's only *raison d'être*.

Consequently, early rather than late referral to palliative care is standard rather than exceptional. Those with cancer, for example, may receive cancer therapy and benefit from palliative care at the same time. This may appear contradictory but a two-pronged approach makes a lot of sense. While chemotherapy and/or radiotherapy targets the cancer, palliative care attends to the unwanted symptoms and, together, they are more likely to improve the quality as well as the length of a person's life. This approach to care is now standard for many other illnesses including AIDS, emphysema and motor neurone disease.

Unfortunately, the old and now mistaken view that palliative care is only for the dying has led many of those with a life-threatening disease, or their family, to decline palliation when it is first offered. Comments like 'I did not know I was that sick' or 'it will frighten Mum (or Dad)' are not unusual and reflect a continuing misunderstanding of contemporary palliative care. The irony is that doctors who make the recommendation are almost certainly practising some form of palliative care at the time and what they seek is specialist advice and not a new approach to care.

In reality, the fear is not with palliative care or what it has to offer, but with what it may signify. The association between palliative care and death is so firmly entrenched in the minds of many people that they believe, in accepting it, they give up on life and resign themselves to death. After becoming ill, many people live in hope of a cure or, if that is not possible, they hope for a life that is not unduly shortened by the disease. So any recommendation for palliative care may be rejected if these hopes (realistic or otherwise) are threatened by outdated beliefs.

My hope is that the health profession and the community will ultimately see palliative care for what it is—a form of care specific to the person rather than the disease; care that bears no temporal relationship to death and where the goal is the achievement of the best possible quality of life. The purpose of palliative care is to help those with cancer or some other incurable illness to live as full and active a life as possible; only when life is clearly drawing to an end does the intent change to facilitating a dignified death.

How it achieves these goals varies from individual to individual. For most it means some form of symptom control— relief of pain, breathlessness, nausea or whatever. In some cases this may be all it involves but, for others, psychological, family, spiritual or existential issues may be just as disabling and require equal attention. No doctor or nurse has the skills to deal single-handedly with the full range of problems that may arise and other members of the palliative care team are frequently called upon to assist. If the problem is pain, a palliative care doctor will be consulted; if it is fear or depression, then a counsellor or social worker is better qualified to advise.

As death approaches, palliative care maintains the emphasis on comfort and seeks also to facilitate a dignified death in the dying person's place of choice. It becomes more available to help with the 'everyday' care, fine-tunes medication, supports the family and friends during this final phase and keeps them informed, as much as is possible, on changes, developments and treatment options. This can be a tense and uncertain time and the daily and often twice daily visits by the doctor and/or nurse can be reassuring and empowering.

Who is eligible for palliative care?

Palliative care was established to deal with the specific and often neglected problems of those with advanced and incurable cancer. In time, cancer patients with less advanced forms of the disease but with equally troublesome symptoms were included and now people with a whole range of illnesses come under the palliative care umbrella. These illnesses include AIDS, lymphoma, leukaemia, motor neurone disease, advanced emphysema, intractable heart problems, liver failure and renal failure where dialysis or transplantation is not possible or declined.

The only eligibility factors for palliative care are:

◆ a progressive illness that is beyond cure or where there is no known cure;

◆ symptoms, be they physical, psychological or spiritual, that are distressing and/or interfere with a person's quality of life;

◆ an expectation that death will ensue as a matter of course.

Are children eligible to receive palliative care?

There is no upper or lower age limit for people seeking palliative care. Children do, however, present special problems and paediatric services usually maintain their involvement when an ill baby or child reaches the palliative stage. Most of the necessary care for these children is provided at home or in hospital-based paediatric units. Only a few capital cities have the specialised units that provide much needed respite for parents and family caring for chronically sick or dying children. Information on these units is available through the state and territory associations or the paediatric service that cares for your child.

Can palliative care be given at home?

Contrary to popular belief, most palliative care is delivered in a person's own home. In Australia today, 30% of people receiving palliative care die at home; the remainder transfer to a palliative care unit, hospital or nursing home days, weeks or months before their death.

A home death is not only desirable but possible. In all but exceptional circumstances, care and comfort is not compromised when someone dies at home. There are, however, some instances when a home death could be problematic. Complex medical problems or carer exhaustion may necessitate admission to a hospital or hospice. A common barrier to a person dying at home is the family's fear and sense of inadequacy in dealing with an emergency, if one should arise. No guarantees can be given that this will not happen but prophylactic measures (see Chapter 4, Managing symptoms other than pain) should ensure the risks are sufficiently low to make home care safe. If this assurance cannot be given, admission may be the preferred option.

When and why are people admitted to a palliative care unit?

Palliative care units are present in most urban and regional centres and eligible subjects (see above) may be admitted for one of the following reasons.

- *Symptom control.* If a symptom is proving difficult to manage at home or if a person requires urgent attention, admission to a specialised palliative care unit is often recommended. The length of stay will depend on the nature of the problem.

- *Respite care.* This type of admission is primarily aimed at giving the carer a break. The admission may be as short as one day or as long as two weeks, depending on the circumstances. During this time the unit provides the ongoing care while the carer catches up on much needed rest, has a holiday or visits family. Respite admissions need to be booked in advance.

- *End-of-life care.* For people who cannot be cared for at home during the final days or weeks of life.

There is no limit to the number of times a person can be admitted for symptom control and respite care but you may find a minimum interval of six weeks or so is imposed between each respite admission.

There may be some difficulties associated with admission to a palliative care unit—distance from the family home and the availability of beds are just two examples. Quite often it is not practical issues but emotional factors that delay or stand in the way of an admission. Your loved one may be afraid they will not see home again or you may be burdened by guilt, fear or anxiety and so resist the admission. These feelings are absolutely normal but should be weighed carefully against the indication for admission and the possible consequences of continuing care at home. Complex medical problems or difficulty in obtaining essential medications can sometimes pose insurmountable barriers for home care. These can be more easily dealt with in a palliative care unit or hospital.

Another reason for carers to resist admission is a promise they may have made to their loved one, often long ago, to continue care at home. Carers feel duty bound to honour this and can be burdened by enormous guilt if admission to a palliative care unit or hospital becomes necessary. It goes without saying, the course of a life-threatening illness is unpredictable and, despite the best intentions, there are times when the burden of care becomes too great. For this reason, a blanket promise to continue care at home is best avoided. A conditional promise that care will continue as long as it is humanly possible and medically reasonable is one that most people understand and accept.

Carer fatigue is a common problem and can be a reason for a planned or urgent admission. If you have reached a point where you can no longer continue, whether for physical or emotional reasons, it is in your and your loved one's interests to acknowledge the need for help and respite. Be very open about your concerns, share them with your loved one and discuss them with the doctor or nurse. You may feel as though you have let your loved one down but, remember, we all have our limits. So do not punish yourself. Recognise the enormous commitment you have already made. The need for transfer can arise despite the best efforts of you and the palliative care team.

If possible, I recommend that you visit the nearest palliative care unit. Seeing the unit at first hand and talking to the staff will dispel fears and allay the anxiety that could otherwise be associated with a future admission. It is desirable to take your ailing relative with you but, if that is not possible, they should at least be informed about the visit and your impressions. Where there is no palliative care unit (as is the case in much of rural Australia), those who cannot be cared for at home are admitted to the nearest public or private hospital. These hospitals may or may not have specialist palliative care personnel but they will have knowledge of palliative care principles and can, if necessary, call the nearest regional service for advice.

There may be reasons why you prefer your loved one to be admitted to a hospital in preference to a palliative care unit. This is particularly true for those who have had a long association with one specialist and one ward. The reassurance that comes with familiar surroundings and personnel makes up for much of the 'busyness' encountered in a hospital and should be taken into account when admission is being planned. Considerable expertise in the care of those with a life-threatening illness is present in both hospitals and palliative care units although the latter offer a more homely environment, have fewer restrictions and are better positioned to care for everyone's needs.

How does a palliative care unit differ from a hospital?

A palliative care unit is not like home nor is it like a hospital. It tends to be smaller, quieter, less hectic and less clinical than the average hospital ward. There are fewer restrictions, hardly any machines, no intravenous drips and none of the usual interruptions such as regular blood pressure or temperature readings. For those used to the hustle and bustle of a hospital, this low-key approach may be seen as casual and one cannot be blamed for thinking the nurses are not doing their job. Quite the opposite! Palliative care strives for a homely approach and, just as care is not compromised at home by the absence of blood pressure or temperature readings, so too within the palliative care unit. Of course, there are times when readings may be taken, tests performed or special treatment given. Palliative care units have the facilities and the expertise for all of this but utilise them only when the need arises.

You may ask how things can be monitored when tests and 'vital signs' are not checked. My answer is, 'You only have to look.' This is the truth and it is what you and I and others do every day. Tests and vital signs rarely tell us things we don't already know or suspect, and then they tell us only about the physical dimension. Those with a life-threatening illness suffer more than the physical complications of an illness and no amount of testing will tell us about their emotional or existential pain. Sitting on the edge of the bed and listening to what is being said is much more valuable than any measurement and gives more information than any investigation. Staff in a palliative care unit may not be engaged in checking 'vital signs' but they are highly focused and attuned to what may be vital for the person occupying the bed.

It is a widely held belief that a palliative care unit is dark and gloomy, full of people who are dying, and is therefore a depressing place for both patients and visitors. There are many sick patients in any palliative care unit, but no more than in a hospital ward. Most of the people are admitted for symptom control or respite and are discharged home rather than die in the unit. Whenever possible, those who are dying are cared for in a single room and are therefore out of the view of other patients and visitors. Surprisingly, it is not the patients who are concerned about deaths in the unit but their relatives. Many of those admitted have by this stage come to terms with the inevitability of death and are not surprised or alarmed by its proximity.

Most palliative care units are not private hospitals. They are usually part of the public hospital system, situated within or near a public hospital. A person may therefore elect to be admitted as a hospital patient, which means there is no associated financial cost. Members of a health fund may choose to be admitted as a private patient but this carries no added privileges such as a single room or the choice of doctor. Specialist palliative care doctors, nurses, volunteers and members of the allied health team who work in that unit provide the necessary care. Your GP or specialist is unable to manage your case but they can visit and make recommendations on treatment.

Many but not all palliative care units in Australia have some affiliation with the Christian tradition. There are usually no visible signs to indicate such a link other than a chapel that serves as a non-denominational place of silence and worship. People of all faiths and those with no formal religious or spiritual beliefs are admitted. All are free and, indeed, invited to have their own minister, priest, rabbi, monk or imam visit, to continue their spiritual practices and perform accepted rituals.

Is a palliative care unit depressing?

This is one of the commonest questions asked about palliative care. It is not an unreasonable inquiry but, in reality, the question carries with it many of the inquirer's own feelings about the nature of the work and death itself. It says as much about their pain as it does about their perception of palliative care.

I have found working in palliative care challenging but extremely rewarding, not only because of what can be done but also because of what I have learnt and continue to learn. But it was not always like that. For three years as a student and a further three years as a doctor I worked in a large Sydney hospital that had its own hospice less than 100 metres away. In all those years I never once visited that hospice or the people within. It seemed a forbidding place and excuses not to visit came easily. I had been trained to save lives and knew those admitted to 'that place' were dying. I would console myself and justify my absence with the thought that there was nothing I could do to help. That was how I rationalised my actions but, if the truth be known, the thought of confronting death on such a large scale was more than I could handle at the time. Like Woody Allen, I preferred to be as far removed from death as possible.

Ironically, I returned to Sydney twenty years later as Medical Director of that same hospice. Much to my surprise and delight the hospice was neither dark nor depressing and the people, although unwell, were more focused on living than many of my non-dying friends. There were certainly times of darkness but, as with nature, brilliant sunshine and rainbows often followed the darkest moments. It had taken twenty years but, true to TS Eliot's words, I now knew the place for the first time.

So, no, a palliative care unit is not depressing but it is not a place for the faint-hearted. I tell doctors who are considering a move into palliative care not even to consider it unless they are prepared to be challenged and to grow. Working at the frontiers with dying people will shake any preconceived ideas about life and death. As a carer and someone very close to the person who is dying, you too will be challenged and often these challenges may seem insurmountable. But just as dawn always follows night, the darkness you find yourself inhabiting will ultimately lift.

This coexistence of light within the darkness finds expression in many ways. One thing that initially surprised me and continues to surprise others is the amount of humour that comes from those who are dying. This may surface in general conversation, during times of reminiscing or as they talk about the future. It may occur as they luxuriate in a spa bath or relax during a foot massage. Much of the humour is dark but it is liberating and gives sick people the opportunity to talk about important things in a lighter vein. There were many times when I did not know whether to laugh or cry. Here are a few examples:

'I wouldn't be seen dead in that outfit!' (referring to clothes
   to be buried in)
'I will die if you say that about me [at the funeral]!'
'I want to look my best when I am dead!'
'Pack my fags just in case…!'
'If you fight like this while I am dying I hate to think what
   you will do when I am dead!' (a mother to her adult
   children)
'Can't you let a man die in peace?' said he when asked to
   have a wash.
'I am going to my Last Supper,' said a woman who was
   being taken to a restaurant by her family.
'If I'm going to die I don't want to eat healthy food—buy
   me a pizza!'

Is palliative care another name for euthanasia?

There is confusion in the minds of many people as to whether
palliative care is just another form of euthanasia. *The Oxford
Dictionary* defines euthanasia as 'a gentle and easy death'
whereas *The Macquarie Dictionary* definition is the *'putting of a
person to death painlessly'*. The latter definition is more in
keeping with euthanasia as we know it, while the former
seems to define palliative care rather than euthanasia.

What does palliative care involve, then, that has some
people accusing it of being nothing less than euthanasia?
Consider the following fictitious scenario: a 50-year-old woman
with advanced cancer of the lung is unconscious and unable to
take anything by mouth. She has previously experienced
considerable pain and required morphine. As she is now
unable to swallow, morphine is given by injection under the
skin to ensure she remains pain-free, but all other tablets are
ceased. An intravenous drip has not been set up but her mouth
and lips are kept moist. She is turned regularly and every effort
is made to maintain her dignity but ultimately she develops a

chest infection. Given the situation, antibiotics are not given and she dies several days later.

Several issues arise from this scenario that have some people, particularly those in the pro-euthanasia lobby, accusing palliative care of practising 'passive' euthanasia. Here I must say something about the use of the terms 'active' and 'passive' when used to describe euthanasia. 'Active' infers a deliberate action and, in the context of euthanasia, this usually involves the administration of a chemical substance with the sole intention of ending a person's life quickly and peacefully. This was the method adopted to end the life of several people with a life-threatening illness when euthanasia was legal in the Northern Territory. 'Passive', on the other hand, implies inaction. Here the intention is not to end life but to avoid or withdraw treatment that is considered futile, but in other situations could be lifesaving. Such treatment may include antibiotics, heart medication, intravenous fluids, artificial feeding or kidney dialysis. The label of 'passive euthanasia' has also been applied to the continued use of medications such as morphine in those who are unconscious or close to death. The accusation made by the pro-euthanasia lobby is that such treatment, although necessary to ensure comfort, may shorten life, even if unintentionally.

These issues lead many to draw similarities between palliative care and euthanasia. I will address each of these issues separately before drawing any conclusion.

Morphine and the question of euthanasia

Pain is a common complication of chronic illness, particularly cancer. Morphine is currently the most effective agent available to relieve this form of pain. The regular administration of morphine prevents pain but does not eliminate the source of pain. If cancer is still present, as it clearly is in those who are dying, pain will reappear if the medication is ceased. Even when unconscious, a person can still perceive pain (see Chapter 6, States of consciousness) and appropriate medication must be continued if pain is to be avoided. In the circumstances, injection is the only option available. The dose given should be the smallest amount required to control the pain but in some cases this may be relatively large. Controversy that has arisen is not because of morphine itself but the use of these larger doses. If morphine is the right drug and the amount administered is the smallest dose that relieves pain, there is no evidence to indicate that this treatment significantly hastens death.

When morphine is given to someone in pain, the danger associated with respiratory depression is virtually non-existent as pain itself is a respiratory stimulant and counteracts any such problem. In contrast, morphine (or heroin) used for recreational purposes and administered directly into a vein greatly increases the risk of respiratory depression and death. This danger lies not so much with the drug itself but with the method of administration. Morphine is rarely if ever administered intravenously in the palliative care situation. If it cannot be given by mouth it is given by injection under the skin (subcutaneous) and the rate of absorption by this route is much too slow to cause serious respiratory depression (see Chapter 3, Living with pain).

I have known many cancer sufferers who required one hundred times the average dose of morphine to control their pain. These individuals were not only pain-free, they were fully conscious, not confused and enjoyed a better quality of life as a result of the treatment. When drowsiness and unconsciousness occur it is usually due to the disease process rather than medication. In some cases, the dose of morphine required to ease pain may induce sleepiness. If this happens and the person has expressed a preference for pain relief over alertness then it would be negligent, unethical and morally wrong to do anything but relieve the pain. The reverse, however, is also true and any person who prefers to remain 'awake' should have their dose reduced until a satisfactory compromise is reached.

Other medications are occasionally implicated in so-called passive euthanasia and the same principles apply as with morphine. The medication involved is given in the smallest dose required to relieve distress and only after the informed consent of the ill person and/or the family.

Cessation of non-essential medication and euthanasia

When someone is dying and has difficulty swallowing, the only medications that are essential are those needed to ensure comfort. To continue other forms of treatment is not only futile, but also impossible once swallowing is impaired. Medications may include tablets for heart trouble, blood pressure or blood clots. The withdrawal of these lessens the burden for the dying person without influencing the outcome or time of death. In my experience, almost every sick or dying person expressed relief when the number of pills they were expected to swallow was reduced.

Intravenous/subcutaneous fluids and euthanasia

This matter is covered in more detail in Chapter 5, Day-to-day care. Intravenous or subcutaneous fluids do not make a dying person feel better (e.g. relieve thirst) and may introduce new problems to the dying process. Fluids may contribute to a person living hours or days longer but whether this justifies their use is not a matter of medical debate but a question of choice for the person concerned and the family.

Withholding antibiotics and euthanasia

Pneumonia is a very common complication in the sick and the elderly, particularly if the person is unconscious or debilitated from the effects of cancer, emphysema or heart failure. It is not unusual in these situations for pneumonia to be the complication that hastens death. That great physician of more than one hundred years ago, Sir William Osler, called pneumonia 'the old man's friend' as it offers a painless and quick release for those dying of old age or chronic illness such as cancer.

One hundred years ago the decision to treat or not treat pneumonia was not so onerous as antibiotics were unavailable. Today we find ourselves in a quandary because we have many powerful antibiotics that can reverse the course of most infections, including pneumonia. When making a decision for or against antibiotics, the overall context and circumstances need to be considered. An antibiotic may improve the pneumonia but an unconscious patient is unlikely to regain consciousness. Quality of life is not improved and treatment may only succeed in prolonging dying. Most reasonable people would agree this is not in a dying person's best interest.

Weighing up the evidence

Allowing people to die with as much comfort and dignity as possible is one of the major goals of palliative care. This inevitably involves the administration of medication to ensure physical comfort and the withholding or withdrawal of treatment that is considered futile. All decisions regarding the initiation or withdrawal of treatment are based on the dying person's known or obtained wishes, or from the family if no such direction is available. This is definitely not active euthanasia, but is it passive euthanasia?

The inevitable conclusion is that there is no such thing as passive euthanasia. Allowing people to die naturally of their disease, free of pain, in a manner of their choosing and with the minimum of interference is not passive euthanasia but good palliative care. Palliative care does not seek to prolong dying nor does it seek to truncate it with medication or other means. The quality of a person's life, the dignity of their dying and a respect for their legitimate choices are the factors that guide the delivery of palliative care.

Palliative care offers a holistic and humane way of caring for someone who is dying. It does not commit dying people to days of deliberate, futile and undignified coma nor to death by dehydration. Palliative care neither hastens nor delays death and seeks only to ease the pain that may be associated with dying. It cannot be held responsible for the times when dying seems unnecessarily prolonged. Good palliative care should ensure that dying people do not suffer but it is often unable to ease the suffering of family and friends, who may consider this manner of life meaningless. It is very difficult for family, friends and carers to sit and watch someone slowly die but, like death, it is an inescapable part of life and not without meaning.

How does palliative care respond to a dying person's request for euthanasia?

A request for euthanasia by a dying person is not only a request for their life to be terminated but also a call for help. To see it simply as a problem that must be solved overlooks the need for that person to talk about the thoughts and emotions that lie behind this thinly disguised cry for help. Any request for euthanasia flag fears and emotions that make death seem more acceptable and less frightening than life itself—fear of suffering, loss of dignity, a sense of hopelessness, uncertainty about the future, the meaningless of their life. Many requests arise because the dying person is ready to die but mistakenly believes treatment is prolonging their dying. Some feel they have become a nuisance and a burden to their family, particularly those responsible for their day-to-day care, and see a quick and painless death as the best solution to the problem.

Because of the many reasons that underlie a request for euthanasia, the best approach is to allow the person to tell their story, to express their fears and concerns and to ensure they are heard. In many, the plea is not that they be killed but that they be allowed to die and that nothing out of the ordinary is done to prolong their life. For a smaller number, the request for euthanasia is real but the opportunity to talk about the reasons and to ventilate their emotions may be sufficient for the moment. There are always a few who persist in their appeal and if it is not met, or if their despair goes unheard, they may attempt suicide or seek help to end their life. The desperation and sense of abandonment these people must feel is unimaginable. On the occasions I have been involved, an opportunity for the person and family to talk seemed to help.

The carer's role in this situation is very difficult. Your feelings and desire to help may become so entangled that you need friends or a counsellor to get through this difficult time. When in doubt, listen to your loved one and to your own heart.

3 Living with pain

Your pain is the breaking of the shell that encloses your understanding.

KAHLIL GIBRAN, *The Prophet*

hen someone receives a diagnosis of cancer their whole world is turned upside down and they are overwhelmed by thoughts and emotions. In the midst of this chaos two thoughts commonly stand out. The first is the possibility the cancer may kill them, and the other is the belief that severe pain will almost certainly accompany their illness. This association between cancer, death and pain is a deeply entrenched belief of most people and makes the mention of the word 'cancer' a death sentence rather than a diagnosis. The fear it invokes is at times a bigger problem than the disease itself, creating enormous personal and family grief and a future that at best remains uncertain. Although pain is not so prominent in other life-threatening illnesses, fear of the unknown and of death are just as real and as damaging as they are with cancer sufferers.

In this chapter I say more about cancer pain and its treatment and explore the ramifications of pain beyond the physical domain. I hope to dispel many of the myths and misconceptions that sometimes stand in the way of effective treatment, resulting in unnecessary pain and hardship. I also look at the concept of suffering, its relationship to pain and how this impacts on those affected. To illustrate the complexity of pain, I begin with a true story that shows how easy it is to overlook someone's suffering when treatment focuses on the disease process rather than the experience of illness in the broader context of life.

Lou was an elderly man with a long and complicated medical history. Late in life he was found to have cancer of the prostate that had already spread to his bones, causing moderately severe pain. As his health deteriorated he went from one specialist to another and despite first-rate medical attention and good pain relief he became very depressed. It seemed this latest illness was robbing him of more than his health. His inability to do the things he loved and his increasing dependence on others led him to believe he was a nuisance, a burden, and better dead than alive. Lou was more afraid of life than death and he now longed to die. This greatly disturbed his family who were unsure how to resolve the dilemma. Lou often sat alone in his workshop and on one occasion his son wandered in and asked what was troubling him. He caught him at a vulnerable time— Lou was more open than usual and told the following story.

There was once a sick elderly man who lived with his only son. One day he said to the son, 'I want you to take me to a place where I can die.' The son knew he was ill but could not understand why he wanted to leave his home. The father gave no explanation and only persisted with his request. Ultimately, the son gave in, not because he wanted him to leave but because he wanted to see what lay behind this odd wish. Because he was so weak, the father asked his son to carry him. After several hours they reached the outskirts of town. When they came to a desolate spot the old man asked that he be left there and told his son to return home. The son was alarmed and insisted they both return home. The old man said, 'You must do as I say, as this is where I carried my father and left him to die.'

A dialogue followed that got to the heart of Lou's depression and ultimately proved to be deeply rewarding and healing. Lou carried an enormous guilt over his own father's death some fifty years earlier and the story he related was an allegory that clearly exposed this long-held grief. Following this disclosure Lou's depression lifted and he was relieved to have shared the pain he had carried all these years. He died shortly after.

The message of this story is so powerful there is no need to elaborate. What is important is that some of the most difficult pains to treat and the ones that are most easily overlooked are those with a non-physical basis. The unveiling of these pains can be as rewarding as the relief of any physical discomfort, with benefits that go beyond belief. Lou broke the shell that had enclosed fifty years of grief and, while the process was painful, the result was liberating. This has had a great impact on my life—Lou was my father and I listened to his story and shared his grief and ultimate healing.

Another point to this story is the danger inherent in 'controlling' something. In Lou's case, specialists managed to control his pain and numerous other medical problems but they did not understand the situation. Despite all their good medicine Lou continued to suffer. His real pain had not been deliberately bypassed but unconsciously overlooked. Control blinds us to what is there before us. It becomes our master, directing our life, keeping us safe and protecting us from things that appear to be painful or uncomfortable. Control protects us, encases our humanity and ultimately limits the ability to feel and to reveal emotions. Left unchecked, it can, like a growing vine, insidiously choke life itself.

 Whatever we seek to control becomes our master.

ELAINE PREVALLET

The benefits that result from understanding (rather than controlling) suffering are reflected in the words of the Dutch philosopher Spinoza, who said, 'Emotion which is suffering ceases to be suffering as soon as we form a clear and precise picture of it.' Many times in this book I speak of the journey people make as they confront their own death and how necessary this may be to their own healing. Lou's healing came not only from him forming a clear and precise picture of his suffering but from sharing it with someone else. And so it is with all forms of healing. You, as family and friends, and we in the health care profession need to be on the lookout for signposts that indicate suffering and to be very careful we do not steer away from them in an effort to control our environment. Marie De Hennezel in her book *Intimate Death* sums this up beautifully: 'There is a need to give shape to one's life and to show this shape, which gives it its meaning, to someone else. Once the telling of it has been accomplished the person seems to be able to let go and die.'

Pain is not just a physical sensation—it is a human experience. The emotions generated by that experience are locked away, but never too far away, and can be reawakened from time to time, often when we are most vulnerable. Human beings have a great capacity for remembering but an even greater capacity for feeling and it is the unlocking and releasing of these thoughts and feelings that often sets someone free.

Pain: what is it?

Pain has been described as an unpleasant sensory and emotional experience that results from some form of damage or injury to tissues within the body. In other words, it hurts (sensory experience) and because it hurts we may cry, call out in anger or, in cases of chronic pain such as with cancer, become depressed (emotional experience). This emotional component is much stronger in those with chronic pain, particularly if the cause of pain also threatens their life.

The overall experience of pain (sensory plus emotional) is not the same for everyone even though the source and intensity of the painful stimulus may be similar. Whether we show pain and the way it is expressed depends on many things other than the source of pain. These include personal and cultural factors, learnt experiences and the circumstances surrounding the pain. Some will endure much pain before they complain while others will exhibit pain behaviour (e.g. cry) even when pain is anticipated.

When someone complains of pain, particularly in the context of cancer, it is helpful to see their pain as the tip of an iceberg; the amount of pain 'showing' depends not only on the underlying disease but on other factors (figure 3.1). As these factors operate below the surface they are easily overlooked but are nonetheless important in the overall expression and treatment of pain. The 'iceberg' concept helps us to see beneath and beyond the visible manifestation of pain and appreciate its wider dimensions.

If the social, emotional and spiritual needs of the person are ignored or if the environment worsens (e.g. becomes noisier), pain may seem worse even when the cause (in this case, cancer) is essentially unchanged. Pain can worsen with the progression of disease but it is important to realise that the overall experience of pain results not just from illness but from a complex interaction of the physical, emotional, social and spiritual state of a person.

As we come to appreciate the complexity of pain, the word itself seems inadequate to convey the broader meaning. Some have described pain as either physical (when it arises from a physical cause) or spiritual (when it has a social, emotional or spiritual basis). This is misleading, as it is not really a question of one form of pain or the other. They nearly always coexist, particularly in a chronic pain situation, and can rarely be separated, although their relative contribution to the manifest pain varies with the situation. The word 'suffering' incorporates the physical and spiritual dimensions of pain and its rawness conveys the undeniable message that we are dealing with a human experience. Suffering rather than pain is more appropriate to the chronic pain situation.

The following sections focus on some of the physical aspects of pain but we should not forget how important the non-physical dimensions are in the expression of pain and suffering. I say more about suffering later in this chapter.

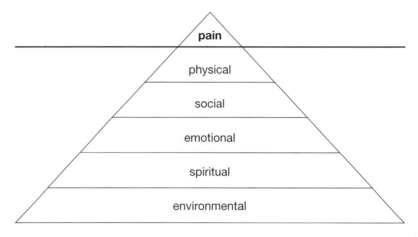

FIGURE 3.1 The 'iceberg' model of pain, showing pain as the tip of the iceberg. How much pain is expressed depends on the presence and magnitude of the factors beneath the surface.

How does cancer cause pain?

Cancer is an abnormal growth of cells within the body. This growth generally begins in one organ and the cancer derives its name from that organ—for example, cancer of the lung means the cancer originated in the lung. Cancers grow and spread locally (lymph glands) and/or to distant organs (liver, bones, brain). As it grows it ultimately compresses and distorts surrounding structures and this results in pain. The amount of pain depends on the degree of pressure and what structures are affected. Pain, for example, is usually worse if bones or nerves are affected.

When cancer spreads from its original site to other organs (e.g. lung cancer that spreads to bone and liver), the cancer in these new sites is still lung cancer. It is not bone cancer or liver cancer. Secondary spread, in medical parlance, is most commonly referred to as a *metastasis* if solitary or *metastases* if multiple. In our example, the correct medical terminology would be cancer of the lung with bone and liver metastases.

Cancer pain is typically chronic and unremitting, and persists for as long as the cancer is present. In the vast majority of cases it responds to conventional pain-relieving medication (analgesics). The pain may worsen over time but can usually be controlled with adjustments in the dose of analgesics. A sudden worsening may indicate some complication and attention will focus on the complication as well as the pain. For example, a fracture will result in a sudden worsening of pain and would be treated like any other fracture with pain relief given at the same time.

Because someone has cancer we should not automatically assume that all pain results from the cancer. Anyone with a serious illness is just as susceptible, often more so, to other painful conditions or complications such as broken bones, shingles, abscesses or cramps. When these are present they are treated in the usual manner, and not simply by increasing the dose of medication. The examples of David and Ashley that follow illustrate this point.

How common is cancer pain?

Contrary to popular belief, pain is not a universal accompaniment of cancer. It is estimated that 50 per cent of people with cancer will have some form of pain or discomfort at time of diagnosis and this will increase to 80–85 per cent as the disease progresses. In other words, up to 20 per cent of those with cancer will be pain-free or relatively pain-free throughout the course of their illness.

Of those that get pain, the majority can expect good to excellent pain relief from conventional medications. A certain proportion, possibly 10 per cent, have pain that is difficult to eradicate and may require larger doses of medication or a combination of several medications to achieve relief. A much smaller number have intractable pain that does not respond or responds only partly to currently available treatment. Unrelieved pain can have devastating effects on an individual, leading in some instances to a sense of hopelessness and despair. Ultimately, this may prove to be as destructive as the pain itself. Alternatively, a complaint of pain may be the only way a person can express the deeper dimensions of their suffering. We must always interpret pain carefully and respond to it appropriately.

Determining the cause of pain

Before deciding on the most appropriate treatment for pain your doctor must exclude treatable and non-cancer causes of the pain. Not all pains are due to cancer and to assume they are may result in inappropriate treatment and could also have serious consequences. For example, a blood clot in the lung not only requires treatment to ease the pain but also specific medication to prevent further clots. The examples of David and Ashley illustrate the importance of determining the exact cause of pain.

David had been in the palliative care ward for several weeks. He had cancer of the lung that had spread to his bones, resulting in considerable pain. The pain slowly improved with analgesics and although not completely pain-free he was able to move around the ward with the minimum of support. One morning he woke with a new and troublesome pain in the right hip. Knowing the cancer had spread to David's bones, the doctor assumed this was the cause of the new pain and ordered an injection of morphine. Before the injection was given the nurse asked the doctor to return to David's bedside to check an unusual finding she had just made. In the bed was a biro top that David had obviously been lying on for some time. This had not only left its mark on his skin but was also responsible for the pain. Once the pen top had been removed, the pain quickly abated.

Ashley had melanoma that had spread throughout his body. One weekend he developed pain in the lower part of his abdomen. Despite an injection of morphine the pain worsened and continued despite two further injections. He was admitted to the local palliative care ward where he was found to have an enlarged bladder. As he was unable to pass urine, a catheter was inserted and a large volume of urine drained, with immediate relief of the pain.

In both examples the pain resolved rapidly once the cause had been determined and appropriate action taken. Neither required analgesics and in Ashley's case the inappropriate use of morphine resulted in unnecessary delay and suffering. Anything other than minor aches and pains needs to be assessed thoroughly before a decision about treatment can be made.

The best assessment involves listening to a person's description of pain followed by a physical examination, taking particular note of body language. It is very difficult to convey to another person the amount of pain we are experiencing. Restlessness, grimaces and unusual positions may say more about a person's pain and its severity than the words they use. Similarly, pain that interferes with sleep or limits activity is strong indirect evidence of severe pain. The opposite also applies and someone who appears comfortable and smiles as they tell you about their pain should make you wonder whether there is more to the pain than a straightforward physical cause. Tests may be required but they should never replace listening and attentiveness. This low-key approach may seem unusual, particularly if tests and technology have occupied a prominent place in your relative/friend's earlier management. Tests will always be done if there is uncertainty about the cause but are not done as a matter of course. They can be burdensome to someone who is unwell and in pain.

Guidelines for the treatment of cancer pain

If analgesics are required to relieve pain, the earlier they are started the better. The pain is easier to control and the dose required to do the job smaller when treatment is not delayed. People do not need to suffer nor do they have to 'earn' their pain relief. If you know or even suspect your relative/friend has pain, encourage them to see a doctor—they may be reluctant to do so for one or more of these reasons:

◆ fear of what may be causing the pain;

◆ fear that death is near;

◆ fear of morphine;

◆ wishful thinking (hoping the pain will go away);

◆ denial (believing the pain is due to something else);

◆ stoicism (accepts the pain is due to cancer but unwilling to have pain relief).

Treatment for pain is given regularly (to prevent pain), not just when pain is present. The dose required over a 24-hour period is generally less and the pain better controlled if medication is given in this way. To take analgesics when there is no pain is a difficult concept to grasp but the logic is simple. Medication suppresses pain but does not get rid of the source of the pain. So, even if medication succeeds in relieving pain, it will certainly return once the medication has washed out of the system. Depending on the medication, this 'washout' time may be as short as 4 hours or as long as 72 hours. The aim is to repeat the medication before the previous dose loses its effect. You will receive clear directions on how this should be done and I recommend you ask the doctor to put all instructions in writing.

Your doctor will always start with a relatively small dose of an analgesic. This minimises side effects but also ensures your relative will get the smallest dose that does the job. The dose will be increased slowly over a matter of days until the pain is relieved. Do not be alarmed if the pain does not settle immediately. It often takes two or three days for the medication to have its full effect after it is commenced and also with every dose increase. If the pain is severe the doctor may start with a slightly higher dose and increase the dose more frequently to achieve rapid control of the pain.

Most analgesics have unwanted side effects so your doctor will advise you on how to overcome these and will prescribe medication if necessary. Constipation is the most common side effect. More is said about side effects later in this chapter and in other chapters.

You will always be given instructions about how to treat an unexpected flare-up of pain. Such pain is called *breakthrough pain* because it has broken through the medication barrier, and the extra medication required to control this pain is called a 'breakthrough'. Approximately two breakthrough doses are permitted in a 24-hour period. If more are required the doctor should be informed as the situation may need to be reassessed. (I suggest you read the following section on morphine and speak to your doctor to ensure you have the necessary medication, and know how and when to use it.)

Call your doctor if there is a sudden worsening or unexpected change in the pain. Whether you do this immediately or later depends on the severity of the pain and the time of day or night. Always err on the side of calling if you are unsure, particularly if pain is severe and has not responded to prescribed breakthrough medication.

ʀadiotherapy and pain control

Radiotherapy utilises high energy X-rays to target the cancer with a view to relieving symptoms (palliative) or to effect a cure (curative). Unfortunately, there are few situations where radiotherapy is curative and more often than not it is used to relieve pain or other distressing symptoms associated with cancer. It does this by shrinking the cancer and thereby relieving pressure on surrounding tissues. It is most effective and most commonly used to ease pain resulting from cancer within the bone. It is also used to shrink cancer in and around vital structures, such as the brain, spinal cord and lung.

When radiotherapy is used to treat pain it is generally given in combination with analgesics as it can take as long as two weeks for the treatment to have its maximum effect. If the person is already taking some form of pain relief the dose may need to be increased during this interim period. The dose of analgesic needs to be reviewed at this two-week mark and the dose reduced, but rarely ceased, if radiotherapy has been effective.

Radiotherapy may be delivered in one or more sessions. The overall health of the person and the site of pain are two of many factors that determine which is preferable. Radiotherapy delivered in one session is obviously more convenient for someone in pain and gives quicker results. Some areas of the body are highly sensitive to radiotherapy and are not suited to this 'one shot' treatment. Treatment to these sites must be given more slowly and over several days. This avoids damage to the surrounding normal tissues without compromising the overall effect on the cancer. The radiotherapy doctor can advise you further on this matter.

Side effects depend on the site to be irradiated and the amount of radiotherapy involved. The larger the dose the greater the risk, and the more central the area of the body to be irradiated the more likely that side effects will appear. Nausea is perhaps the most common side effect and, if anticipated, can be prevented by pretreatment with suitable medication. Redness of the skin and inflammation of mucosal surfaces (mouth, oesophagus) may also occur. The radio-therapy department will always let you know if side effects are expected and will willingly discuss any aspect of the treatment with you. Information booklets are also available from the radiotherapy department and these give more detail on treatment and its effects.

Analgesics and pain control

If pain is troublesome or persistent, pain-relieving medication (analgesics) will almost certainly be sought by the sufferer or recommended by the doctor. As much as we seek relief from pain, the introduction of analgesics often raises questions and concerns that need to be addressed. These concerns are greatest if morphine is the recommended medication, particularly if this is the first time the dreaded 'M' word has been used. Most people associate its use with impending death or believe it may hasten death. These are just two of the many myths and misconceptions that are addressed later in this chapter.

The number and range of pain medications available have increased dramatically in recent years. Many of them are not new but have been resurrected as palliative care and pain control become an increasingly important part of health care. Morphine is still the most effective and most commonly used analgesic for cancer pain relief, but a review of other frequently prescribed analgesics follows.

Commonly used analgesics

◆ **Paracetamol**, better known as Panadol or Panamax, is frequently used in the palliative care situation to relieve pain. Although it is a weak analgesic and recommended for the relief of minor pains, paracetamol can potentiate the effect of other analgesics such as morphine. In other words, if used with morphine the combination is better than morphine alone and may allow a reduction in the morphine dose. This advantage is not only in pain relief; any reduction in the dose of morphine reduces the likelihood of side effects. There is, however, one significant disadvantage. This synergistic effect often requires a minimum of 6–12 paracetamol tablets/day and these, on top of other medication, may be more than a sick person can swallow.

♦ **Aspirin**. While paracetamol has some value in the relief of cancer pain the same cannot be said for aspirin. Aspirin is as good an analgesic as paracetamol but it 'thins the blood' and this can increase the risk of bleeding in someone with cancer. This blood-thinning property is used to advantage in those with heart or circulation problems but is potentially risky and therefore not used in cancer.

♦ **Panadeine Forte**. This combination of paracetamol and codeine is a much stronger analgesic than paracetamol but significantly weaker than morphine. It is extremely constipating and this limits its usefulness, as does the large number of tablets that must be taken to achieve pain relief.

♦ **Tramadol** is a relatively old drug that has only recently been introduced into Australia. It is as effective as Panadeine Forte but has the advantage of being less constipating. It is available in short-acting and long-acting tablet form and is relatively effective in mild to moderate pain.

♦ **Oxycodone** is also known as Endone or Oxynorm (short-acting form) or Oxycontin (long-acting form). It is reputed to be as effective as morphine but a major disadvantage is the lack of a readily available injectable form that can be used if swallowing becomes a problem. Oxycodone has the same pattern of side effects as morphine and is a good alternative for those with moderate to severe pain or those who wish to avoid morphine.

♦ **Fentanyl** is perhaps the newest of the analgesics for relief of cancer pain. Its main advantage is that it is applied to the skin as a patch and only needs to be changed every 72 hours. It is therefore very convenient and easy to use. It appears to be less constipating than most other analgesics and is not as sedating as morphine. It is not recommended when pain is unstable or severe and is inferior to morphine in providing comfort or allaying anxiety around the time of death. It is nonetheless a very useful and frequently prescribed analgesic.

- **Hydromorphone** (also known as Dilaudid) is a very old drug that has recently been reintroduced into the Australian market for treatment of cancer pain. It is a very good analgesic but no better than morphine. Its main use to date has been with people who are unable to tolerate morphine.

- **Methadone** is a very good but underused analgesic. It has a complex metabolism and this has limited its use. As palliative care doctors become more familiar with its idiosyncrasies it will be used more, particularly for 'nerve' pain or for those people unable to tolerate the more commonly used analgesics.

- **Heroin**. A section of the community believes heroin is a better analgesic than morphine and should be made available for those with cancer pain. Heroin is simply two morphine molecules joined together and once in the body is changed immediately into morphine. It is therefore morphine by another name. Heroin is not available for medical use within Australia.

- **Pethidine** is frequently used when pain is transient (rather than chronic), as with trauma or following surgery. It is not recommended nor should it be used when pain relief is required over a prolonged period as is the case with cancer or other forms of chronic pain. Pethidine has a brief duration of action and potentially toxic breakdown products that can accumulate with continuous use. For these reasons it is rarely if ever used in palliative care.

- *Marijuana*. There is not a lot of convincing evidence to show that marijuana helps with cancer pain. I have had many patients who swear by it, but in most cases they had been recreational users well before the time of their illness.

I believe there are many better options for treating pain but can understand why people may want to try marijuana in painful or life-threatening situations, with or without more conventional analgesics.

◆ **Morphine** is the oldest and still the best drug to treat cancer pain. It is the analgesic most doctors use in a palliative care situation because of its effectiveness, relative safety and ease of use. As with most strong analgesics it does have side effects, the most important being constipation. This problem is so common and potentially distressing that laxatives are always prescribed at the same time.

Morphine is available in numerous strengths and in short-acting and long-acting forms. It comes as a liquid, tablet and capsule and also as an injection. This large variety of strengths and forms allows your doctor to fine-tune the dose of morphine to the level of pain and to use the smallest dose necessary. Because of this range, the dose may be increased by changing the strength of the medication rather than increasing the number of tablets. This is a big advantage for someone already taking a large number of pills.

The quick or short-acting form (liquid morphine) is used when someone is first given morphine because it allows for quick and effective control of pain and easier titration of the dose against pain. Because of its rapid action (20 minutes after swallowing) liquid morphine is also used to treat breakthrough pain—that is, pain that appears despite the regular use of pain medication. Liquid morphine has a bitter taste but this can be largely overcome by mixing it with apple juice or other drinks, preferably not alcohol.

The long-acting forms of morphine come in tablet or capsule form and are usually substituted for liquid morphine once pain has been controlled and the dose relatively stable. The most commonly used preparations are MS Contin and Kapanol. Unlike the liquid form, these preparations may take several hours to reach their maximum effect so their effectiveness depends on them being taken regularly and exactly as prescribed. Their slow onset of action also makes them unsuitable for breakthrough pain. The long-acting tablets and capsules must be swallowed whole and not chewed. If there is difficulty swallowing, a long-acting morphine suspension is available. Alternatively, the contents of the morphine capsule can be sprinkled onto ice cream or yoghurt and then swallowed.

Morphine myths and misconceptions

 One fears only what one does not understand.

ANTON CHEKHOV

The perception most people have of morphine can be likened to the reputation that many of our politicians unfairly acquire simply because their actions are often misunderstood. Morphine's poor reputation is based on myths and misconceptions that have their origins in the abuse and misuse of the drug rather than its measured and predictable effects. Because it is categorised as a drug of addiction it is held to be as dangerous as any of the 'street drugs' and is thus guilty by association. Fear of addiction has always been a concern. But of even greater concern among those with cancer and other life-threatening illnesses is that the introduction of morphine heralds the beginning of the end. Offering someone morphine for pain is almost equivalent to proclaiming their imminent death and its introduction is often resisted for this reason.

If strongly held, these views can delay the introduction of effective pain relief and contribute to unnecessary suffering. Sadly, it is the family rather than the person in pain that has most difficulty with morphine and frequently resists the mere mention of the word. This resistance has as much to do with the family's grief as it has with any misconception, and attention to this can often result in a change of heart as well as a change of mind.

The following questions and answers may clarify some of the concerns you have about morphine, improve your understanding of its use and remove some of the associated fear.

Is morphine addictive?

Yes and no. If morphine is administered directly into the vein for a sufficiently long period it may result in addiction. Given in this way, morphine, like many other drugs, produces an immediate euphoria and it is this that makes it potentially addictive. Morphine (or any analgesic) is rarely if ever administered into the vein in a palliative care situation. It is nearly always given by mouth as a tablet, capsule or liquid or as an injection under the skin. Absorption is much too slow by either of these routes to induce euphoria and so the risk of addiction is virtually zero. Caution must be exercised in those who have previously been addicted to morphine, heroin or some other drug. Even then morphine can be used safely and effectively but its administration does require special care.

If morphine is started early will it work when it is really needed?

Morphine will continue to work for as long as it is given. If the dose required increases over time this is because the pain has worsened, not because the person has developed a tolerance to its effect. It is not unusual for palliative care patients to be on morphine for months or years and even over this length of time tolerance does not develop.

Does starting morphine now mean the end is near?

Morphine is recommended for the relief of pain or other symptoms and may be required very early in the illness or at some later stage. In the past, morphine was reserved for those close to death but that was before its safety and usefulness was fully appreciated. It is too good a drug to be reserved for special occasions. It is the best and safest drug for the treatment of pain (and other symptoms) and that is why doctors advocate its use early rather than late in the illness.

Can morphine be used for symptoms other than pain?

Morphine is very effective in relieving cough or easing the distress associated with breathlessness. The dose required for these symptoms is often, but not always, less than that used for pain.

Is morphine safe?

Any drug, morphine included, must be used with due care. Morphine is a remarkably safe drug, particularly when given by mouth or injection under the skin, which are the routes most frequently used in palliative care. Given in this way, it will not shorten the length of time a person lives. Reports of morphine killing or being used to kill someone always involve inappropriately large doses given directly into the vein. Such a risk applies to any drug, not just morphine.

Is it safe to use morphine for long periods?

Morphine can be used safely and effectively for quite long periods. The fact that it is recommended and approved by statutory bodies for the treatment of chronic pain due to causes other than cancer speaks volumes for its safety.

Is morphine safe when given in large doses?

Those with severe pain are very likely to require a large dose of morphine. The large dose will be arrived at over a period of time and this slow escalation generally reduces the likelihood of unacceptable side effects. The risk of drowsiness does increase with dose and this may be a problem for some. Used carefully and correctly, morphine is absolutely safe even in large doses—the biggest worry is the underlying illness that creates the need for such big doses.

Is there anything else that can be used in place of morphine?

Many drugs can be used to treat cancer pain. None is better, safer or more effective than morphine. Apart from paracetamol, they are all closely related to morphine and have similar side effects. Morphine is recommended because of its safety and effectiveness and because it is a tried and tested analgesic. Anything weaker may not have the desired effect. Analgesics of equivalent strength have no added advantage but are used for the occasional person who cannot tolerate morphine.

What would make you think an alternative analgesic is necessary?

The most common reason for withdrawing morphine and substituting another analgesic is a side effect that cannot be prevented or overcome by a dose reduction. These side effects may include nausea, vomiting, drowsiness, confusion, intractable constipation and itch.

Does a history of morphine allergy mean it cannot be used?

Morphine allergy is extremely rare. Most people are told they are allergic because of vomiting that followed an injection, often after an operation. This is not an allergy, but almost certainly a side effect of the morphine or the operation. It does not preclude further use of morphine although the doctor will almost certainly use anti-vomiting medication in the face of such a history. In the rare case of true morphine allergy, morphine should be avoided and one of the other analgesics used in its place.

Does morphine cause drowsiness?

Like many other drugs, morphine can result in some drowsiness when first commenced or if the dose is increased. This drowsiness generally improves after a few days, but if it does not the dose may be reduced. If that is not possible (because of pain) an alternative analgesic may be tried.

Does morphine cloud the mind?

The larger the dose of morphine the more likely it is to cloud the mind. Large doses are used only for severe pain, which if untreated or inadequately treated will itself cloud the mind and impair function much more than morphine ever would.

What other side effects occur apart from drowsiness?

The most common side effects are dry mouth and constipation. Frequent sips of fluid are recommended for the former and laxatives will be required to prevent the latter. Other side effects include vomiting (already mentioned), itching, sweating, confusion and muscle twitches. Confusion is very uncommon but if it does occur the dose of morphine may need to be reduced. Failing that, morphine may be ceased and an alternative analgesic given. Muscle twitching is generally of nuisance value and tends to occur as one is falling asleep. If severe, the dose of morphine should be reduced, pain permitting.

Will side effects occur with other analgesics if they have already occurred with morphine?

It is possible but the risk is less. Occasionally, the doctor may have to trial several analgesics before the best and least troublesome one is found. It is certainly better to try an alternative than leave someone in pain.

Can a person drive a motor vehicle or continue working while taking morphine?

Driving a car is permitted providing the person is on a stable dose of morphine, not drowsy and deemed to be safe on all other accounts—for example, not too weak. Following any dose increase the person should cease driving for a few days, until the effect of that increased dose becomes apparent. Much the same applies to work when safety issues are involved. The RTA should be advised about the use of morphine and, subject to the above provisos, problems rarely arise. The driving of larger passenger vehicles or trucks is another matter and this needs to be discussed with your doctor.

Can morphine be ceased after it has been commenced?

Just because the pain has improved does not mean there is no further need for morphine. More often than not the pain is better because the medication is keeping it at bay. Stopping the morphine will almost certainly result in a rapid and dramatic resurgence of pain. So never stop morphine without discussing it with the person overseeing its use. In the uncommon situation where the pain does disappear, the morphine dose may be reduced slowly, but this must be done carefully and under medical supervision.

Why can't morphine be withdrawn abruptly?

If a person has been taking morphine for some time, stopping it suddenly can result in unpleasant symptoms like restlessness, insomnia and sweating. This is a physical withdrawal and not due to addiction. The same withdrawal occurs with other commonly prescribed medications and even with tea or coffee. Addiction is said to be present when a person craves for a drug and the craving results in antisocial behaviour.

Does this mean morphine has to be taken for the rest of a person's life?

Morphine may need to be taken for the rest of a person's life— not because of withdrawal symptoms but because the pain that occurs with cancer usually persists and unfortunately worsens rather than improves with time. If for some reason the pain does disappear and morphine is withdrawn, this will be done slowly.

Is morphine a dangerous drug?

No more dangerous than any other drug but, as with all drugs, it should be kept in a safe place and certainly out of the reach of children.

How and where should morphine be stored?
Morphine is best stored in a safe, cool place, and out of direct sunlight.

Are there any non-drug measures that can be tried to improve pain?
Hot packs may be useful in the treatment of pain but must be used carefully to avoid skin damage or burns. Massage, therapeutic touch and meditation have also been shown to help. Acupuncture and TENS (transelectrical nerve stimulation) also have a place. TENS is similar to acupuncture in its effect but utilises low levels of electrical current in place of needles. All these non-drug measures may ease minor pains but rarely improve cancer pain. They are often used in combination with morphine for some of the more troublesome pains, not as an alternative.

Does morphine relieve any of the suffering that may accompany pain?
If the suffering is partly or wholly due to chronic or severe pain, treatment of the pain will significantly improve physical comfort and morale. Morphine, however, does not improve other forms of suffering and if increasing doses are mistakenly used for emotional or spiritual pain the situation may worsen. As with any pain, the exact cause must be found and appropriate treatment instituted. Sometimes, this treatment may simply entail listening.

Resistant pain

This is one of the most difficult scenarios in palliative care. Unrelieved pain robs a person of quality time and may ultimately lead to despair and a sense of hopelessness. Family and friends are not spared, as they look on helplessly, wondering what can be done to relieve their relative/friend's suffering. Treatment of resistant pain is an emergency, not only because of the pain but also to counteract the untold emotional harm that can result if the situation continues for any length of time.

In most cases, pain relief comes from using larger doses of morphine. While this may be effective, it introduces a whole new set of problems, the main one being drowsiness. Whether this is preferable to pain is a personal matter and, for this to be an informed decision, a trial of a bigger dose may be necessary. The ultimate dose required to control the pain may be large, but gradual increases rather than a sudden escalation allows adequate time to assess the beneficial effect and side effects on a daily basis. As long as the benefits outweigh the disadvantages the plan of increasing the dose remains reasonable, but the final decision is always in the hands of the person receiving the treatment or their delegate.

The dose required to achieve the desired outcome is sometimes extraordinarily high and may be up to one hundred times the average dose. Side effects may be surprisingly few, but drowsiness and confusion are the most frequent and cause the most concern. Drowsiness may or may not be acceptable but confusion never is. If confusion is thought to be due to morphine, a dose reduction rather than complete withdrawal may be all that is required. If this compromises pain relief the doctor will almost certainly recommend another analgesic in place of morphine.

You may hear or read reports that suggest large doses of morphine can hasten death by depressing respiration, thereby implying that this approach to pain relief is nothing short of euthanasia. These reports are misleading and alarmist and create unnecessary anguish for all concerned. Morphine used correctly to relieve pain does not hasten death. If you are worried about this, speak to the most senior doctor involved in your relative/friend's care and discuss the matter fully.

Pain relief comes at a cost, particularly if alertness is compromised. If this is the course chosen by the person in pain, anything less would be inhumane and unethical. People like Tom (see Introduction) may value alertness over pain relief and for them drowsiness would not be acceptable and compromises must be made.

Dawn had multiple myeloma, a malignancy that softens bones and increases the likelihood of fractures. She had several fractured ribs as a result of coughing. This caused considerable pain, particularly on movement. The only relief was from morphine but the dose required for relief resulted in drowsiness. Dawn chose to remain alert and only asked for 'extra' morphine at night to help with sleep, or during the day when the pain was particularly severe.

She knew she was dying but as there were several family rifts she chose to remain as alert as possible, hoping to heal these divisions. Despite the pain and discomfort she organised family meetings and presided over sessions that not only brought healing to the warring parties but to herself also. When this was completed she requested larger doses of morphine to ease the pain. The dose was increased until she was comfortable at rest and only experienced mild discomfort with turning and movement. She was drowsier than before but was still able to maintain meaningful contact with her family until several days before her death.

Times like these can be particularly hard. Accepting the death of someone you love is hard enough but to witness suffering in the form of unrelieved pain, or to be asked to make compromises for the sake of pain relief, is often more than anyone can bear. If this is true for you, find someone you can talk to, someone who can hear your story without feeling they must solve it. If you have misgivings about the way your loved one's pain is being treated, ask for a meeting with the doctor(s) and nurses, let them know of your concerns and seek clarification about the treatment plan, now and in the future. This may not ease your immediate pain but advocating for your relative and taking positive steps to deal with uncertainty removes some of the helplessness that can otherwise overwhelm. It is the 'not knowing' that causes the most harm. The treatment of resistant pain may be problematic but there is always something that can be done. This 'something' may fall short of complete pain relief or may introduce new problems. Despite these shortcomings, the knowledge that there are treatments that can improve pain goes a little way towards restoring hope.

Before outlining the options available for the treatment of resistant pain I must stress that these alternatives are rarely used at the start. They are considered only after morphine and/or other analgesics have been given a fair and adequate trial. Treatment that may be acceptable for one person may not suit another and so choices are always negotiated and treatment individualised.

◆ Certain drugs other than conventional analgesics may help with resistant pain. These medications are grouped under the name 'co-analgesics' and alone or together with morphine they may improve certain types of pain, especially nerve pain. These drugs include cortisone, ketamine (a very old anaesthetic agent) and medication commonly used to treat conditions such as depression, epilepsy or heart troubles.

◆ A change in the type of analgesic may be recommended as each works a little differently. So, if morphine has not been effective or is associated with intolerable side effects, another may give better results.

◆ A spinal infusion is occasionally recommended. Drugs such as morphine can be delivered via this system directly into the spinal cord where they act to relieve pain. Delivering morphine directly to the point at which it acts allows a much smaller dose to be used than that required by mouth or injection. As the dose is smaller, side effects like drowsiness are considerably less. Despite this theoretical advantage, spinal infusion for resistant pain has mixed results. It works well for some but not for others. Careful selection is the key to its success.

◆ In the very unusual situation where pain persists despite the above measures there is the option of using sedation combined with morphine to control pain. Sedation does not eliminate pain but, as the person sleeps more, they are less aware of pain. This is a very complex situation and the use of sedation to ease pain has significant legal, moral and ethical implications. I have used it rarely and only after all other forms of pain relief have failed and where the person has sought pain relief. Family members often found the choice much harder to accept and derived little comfort from seeing their relative more asleep than awake, even though pain-free. Whether this is a form of euthanasia has been hotly debated for many years. We do tread a fine line when we embark on this path but there are few alternatives when someone is dying in pain, and for those people it is pain rather than death they most fear.

Suffering

Embrace sadness lest it turn to despair.

MICHAEL LEUNIG

What better way to introduce the subject of suffering than through the portal of intractable pain? The two are so inextricably linked we cannot contemplate treatment of one without some understanding of the other. Disease processes affect not only our body but our essential being and it is this disruption and threat to life that contributes to human suffering.

What is suffering? It is an intense feeling and like all feelings is almost beyond words. Suffering is as hard to describe as joy, love, hatred or despair and has to be felt to be fully understood. And just as a smile, a cry or a laugh is unique to every individual so too is suffering. We may have some appreciation of other people's suffering but that appreciation stems from our experience rather than theirs and is at best distorted. This is a lesson I learnt very early in my palliative care career.

Harry was readmitted to the hospice for what I knew would be his last visit. He had pneumonia and was semi-conscious at the time. He had been in and out of hospitals and hospices over the preceding few years because of a cancer that had by now eaten away the centre of his face. This large cavity was covered by an artificial nose and what that did not cover was hidden by a mask. No amount of camouflage could disguise the smell and I could only imagine the amount of suffering Harry must have felt and the barriers this cancer created.

Harry died and after his death I spoke to his wife and said, somewhat thoughtlessly, that his suffering was now over. Her reply was quick and forgiving as she lovingly pointed out that his suffering was not as bad as I had imagined. She said that he was happy as long as he could have a drink and place a bet and had not for one moment wished for death.

What Harry's case suggests is that we don't *feel* other people's suffering but only *imagine* what it would be like if we were in the same position. Some people call this empathy and, while empathy gives us a feel for what it might be like for someone, we should accept that it often falls short of the mark. Suffering is what it means for that person, and the best way for us to get to know the extent and nature of other people's suffering is to allow them to talk about it.

Many attempts have been made to define suffering and these lines from *The Prophet* come close to describing this unique human experience: 'When you are sorrowful, look again in your heart, and you will see that in truth you are weeping for that which has been your delight.' This suggests that sorrow or suffering arises not simply because of some situation that we find ourselves in but because of what it deprives us of. We suffer because of what we have lost or are about to lose.

We know sorrow (suffering) because we have known delight. And therein lies the source of the pain. Memories bring joy to a dying person but they are also the source of much suffering as they remind them of what was and may never be again. Suffering is therefore almost inevitable in the context of dying. It cannot be ignored nor can the dying person be shielded from it. There is no cure, or any trick or medicine that makes it better. It is only by entering into the suffering and feeling its tight embrace that the dying person eventually finds a way through. As Michael Leunig suggests, to ignore suffering leads to despair.

What can you do then, as a carer, if you see or feel your loved one's suffering? The answer may seem simple but is much harder than it sounds. When the moment arrives, allow them to talk and experience their sorrow. Don't reassure, console, change the subject, answer a ringing phone or find some reason to leave the room. Just be there for them. By doing this you give them permission to open their heart, feel what is inside and get to know what is being revealed. Only through experiencing their suffering is healing likely to occur.

The moment cannot be contrived—it will occur spontaneously, often without good reason, but a seemingly minor thing like a phone call, photograph, favourite tune or a memory may be the stimulus for the outpouring. This spontaneous confession connects the person to the language of their heart and not their head and this is exactly where you want them to be. If they are in their head they may be able to talk about their suffering but unless they experience it there will be no catharsis or healing. Asking questions is one sure way of getting them out of their heart and into their head, so don't feel as though you need to speak or make things better. Silence as always is golden.

Don't be deceived into thinking your role in all this is just one of a spectator. Your presence creates the space that allows all this to happen. It is as if you hold the light that allows your loved one to find their way. And while your loved one is likely to feel better for having let go of some of their suffering, you may need a friend or counsellor with whom you can debrief and let go of some of your own pain. As this catharsis usually occurs in episodes rather than one big performance, friends become a necessity rather than a luxury.

4 Managing symptoms other than pain

The value of life, like all things precious, is often felt most when damaged or discarded.
Regardless of the carnage it is always worthy of repair
and whilst forever altered,
what was once precious is now priceless beyond compare.

ANON

*t*ime is precious for someone who is dying but it is the quality of that person's life that determines how precious a commodity it is. The term 'quality of life' has become something of a cliché but most would agree that bodily comfort is an essential, if not the most essential, ingredient. Those of you who have gasped for air or experienced severe pain or intractable vomiting will appreciate how symptoms like these can undermine the quality of life. It is not unusual to hear someone in such a situation say 'I wish I could die'. We know this is not to be interpreted literally but the comment says a lot for how bodily discomfort impacts on life.

For most of us, the problem is usually transient. We are so grateful when it is over and go to any lengths to avoid a repeat performance. The thought that it may recur can fill the strongest person with fear. If this is true, spare a thought for those with a life-threatening illness where symptoms are equally distressing and rarely transient, and where the prospect for cure is all but non-existent. A life of pain (by 'pain' I mean any form of physical distress) can fill the sanest and strongest person with despair.

You may be thinking this is all a bit of an exaggeration—but is it? To live in intractable pain, with constant nausea or unremitting breathlessness not only robs people of quality of life, it robs them of valuable time and of life itself. This chapter shows that it is not necessary for anyone with a life-threatening illness to endure physical distress. We may not be able to cure the underlying disease but a lot can be done to palliate the symptoms common to most diseases. In so doing, we do not prolong life but restore some of the value attached to life.

The emphasis in this chapter is on cancer and its associated symptoms but what is said in relation to care and treatment can be applied to most life-threatening illnesses. However, some treatments that are quite specific for cancer (e.g. radiotherapy) are not applicable to other illnesses. In most cases, this will be obvious but, where it is not, explanations are given.

The nature and range of symptoms associated with advanced cancer vary enormously and depend mainly on the cancer's site of origin and the degree of spread. As a general rule the number and severity of symptoms increase as the cancer grows, but this is not always true. For example, pain may be as severe with a small, localised cancer as it is with widespread disease; alternatively, a person may have widespread disease and yet remain remarkably free of symptoms. Much the same applies to any life-threatening illness.

Symptoms are not always due to the disease process and those who have trod the cure path will know all too well the potential problems associated with medications like chemotherapy. But it is not only chemotherapy that causes problems. Simple medications such as antibiotics and laxatives can produce more than their fair share of trouble. Symptoms may arise for any number of reasons and your doctor will always look for a cause before making any suggestions about treatment.

Looking for a cause may involve blood tests and/or X-rays

but a good history and physical examination often suffice. So do not be alarmed if the doctor does not order tests. Tests are invasive and involve some degree of hardship; for those who are unwell tests are reserved for situations where the origin of the symptom(s) is not clear-cut. This 'softly, softly' approach may be in stark contrast to what your relative/friend experienced in the early stages of their illness. It does not imply lack of care but rather a more holistic approach to care.

It also worth remembering that the person with cancer is not a mere passenger in their illness but responds in ways that say as much about their emotional and spiritual state as about the disease itself. This aspect of care must not be overlooked and I hope it has been covered sufficiently in other chapters for you to appreciate its importance. Concentrating solely on what is happening on the 'outside' may lead us to overlook what is happening on the 'inside', and the relief of symptoms is therefore only part of the overall care. In all forms of care, attention should always be on the whole person and not just the part that 'pains'.

 You can be absolutely brilliant without knowing what is going on.

WOODY ALLEN

Breathlessness

In the context of palliative care this symptom is most frequently seen in those with advanced disease of the heart or lungs, cancer of the lung or any cancer that has spread to the lung. The resulting damage or destruction interferes with normal gas exchange and a person must breathe faster and more deeply to get sufficient oxygen. It is this need to breathe 'harder' that results in the sense of breathlessness.

The distress associated with breathlessness should never be

underestimated. It can be very frightening, particularly during sudden or severe exacerbations, so much so that the person may think they are about to die. Even though it is a highly visible symptom the degree of distress may be difficult to assess, for any number of reasons. So always rely on what your loved one says and, if you are uncertain, err in their favour and if necessary ask your doctor or palliative care nurse to assess the situation.

Irrespective of the cause, breathlessness may be aggravated by a number of factors including a chest infection, anaemia or fluid that accumulates around the lungs (pleural effusion). The appropriateness and value of antibiotics in treating a chest infection will depend on circumstances more than the nature of the infection. As a general rule, the sicker the person and the closer they are to death the less likely antibiotics are to help. Having said this, the decision for or against antibiotics is never easy, particularly if some form of an advanced directive has not been given.

While experience has shown that treatment for anaemia, including transfusion, rarely results in any significant improvement, drainage of pleural effusion may give worthwhile albeit temporary relief. The procedure is not without risk and the decision for or against drainage should be made only after discussion and careful consideration of the potential risks and likely benefits. The wishes of the person, their state of health, the severity of the symptom and the amount of fluid present are the factors most likely to influence that final decision. Drainage can only be done in a hospital or hospice, is performed under local anaesthetic and, depending on the size of the effusion, may take as long as one hour to complete.

General measures to help breathlessness

◆ Those who are breathless generally prefer a well ventilated room. A stuffy, overheated room can make them feel worse even if it does not make breathing harder. Open windows and/or a fan may help, but the final say should be left to the one you are trying to help.

◆ Home oxygen is not always necessary but the option should be discussed with the doctor early in the course of the illness. If oxygen is recommended, your doctor or community nurse will make the necessary arrangements for its delivery and they or the supplier will show you how to use the equipment. I say more about oxygen shortly but, on a practical note, oxygen concentrators (but not cylinders) are available free of charge to those who belong to a palliative care program.

◆ Plan ahead so that activities that induce breathlessness, such as showering and toileting, don't occur at the same time.

◆ Ten minutes of oxygen before and during exertion can be helpful. If oxygen is used continuously, increasing the rate of flow does not help as much as a planned, assisted and unhurried approach to activities.

◆ Take whatever measures are necessary to prevent consti-pation as this sets up a vicious cycle where constipation aggravates breathlessness and breathlessness in turn makes it harder to deal with constipation.

Oxygen

Oxygen may be a lifeline for those who are breathless, and when required is administered via nasal prongs or a mask. Nasal prongs is usually the better and preferred option. It interferes less with eating, is not as claustrophobic as a mask and poses less of a barrier to communication. Oxygen is run at 2 litres/minute or thereabouts when given via nasal prongs and 4–5 litres/minute by mask. Increasing the rate of oxygen delivery does not give a proportionate improvement in breathlessness, but a higher flow rate is advisable in severe cases or with acute exacerbations.

The most common means of delivering oxygen is an oxygen concentrator. This is an electrically operated device that extracts oxygen from the atmosphere and concentrates it for subjects to breathe. When in operation a concentrator makes a constant droning noise, which some people find quite irritating. This problem is easily overcome by placing the concentrator in another room and running a long connection from it to the nasal prongs or mask. Unlike an oxygen cylinder, a concentrator provides an endless supply of oxygen but can only deliver a maximum of 5 litres/minute. Running at this rate for a prolonged period can overwork the machine and result in mechanical problems. Oxygen via nasal prongs can be very drying to the nose but this can be lessened by keeping the flow rate at 2 litres/minute or by applying vaseline to the nostrils. If both these measures fail, a humidifier, available from the oxygen supplier, will moisten the inspired oxygen and overcome the problem.

If oxygen is required at a rate exceeding 5 litres/minute, two concentrators run in parallel can deliver up to 8 litres/minute. Oxygen can be given at much higher rates (up to 10–12 litres/minute) via a cylinder, but the hiring and replacement costs of cylinders and the associated logistics make this a less attractive alternative. The concentrator is usually the preferred option. It is easy to use, very effective and the 'quality' of the oxygen it delivers is as good as that from a cylinder.

People often ask whether an oxygen cylinder should be kept in reserve in case of mechanical or electrical failure. As concentrators are very reliable and blackouts uncommon, a backup supply of oxygen is recommended in only a small number of cases. The severity of the breathlessness and the degree of oxygen dependence are the two major factors in this decision. If you are concerned, discuss the matter with your doctor. While backup cylinders are rarely required, a small 'portable' cylinder may be useful for short outings in a car or wheelchair that might otherwise not be possible.

Do remember that oxygen is highly inflammable and should not be used near an open flame or where sparks may occur. Smoking is, of course, not permitted in the same room or anywhere nearby.

Morphine

Morphine is commonly used to treat breathlessness. This may come as a surprise but morphine and oxygen are the two most effective agents available for the treatment of this distressing symptom. Morphine is generally given by mouth and experience suggests the liquid (quick-acting form) is more effective than the slow-release tablet or capsule. If the breathlessness is not too bad, the convenience of taking a tablet or capsule twice daily may influence your doctor to recommend the slow-release form in preference to liquid. As with pain, morphine is always given regularly rather than intermittently; extra or breakthrough doses may be required if there is a sudden worsening of the symptom (see Chapter 3, Living with Pain, for further details on breakthrough morphine). The dose of morphine can be increased for worsening breathlessness just as it is for worsening pain.

Research is currently being done to see whether morphine via a nebuliser is as effective as that given by mouth. The jury is still out on this—most agree it is no more effective but side effects may be fewer. Despite this, most doctors still favour the oral route, not only because it is simpler but also because the absorption and therefore the action of the morphine is more predictable. If the nebulised route is chosen, be aware it is the injectable morphine that is used in the nebuliser, not the liquid or oral form.

Some doctors are a little hesitant about using morphine to treat breathlessness if it is partly or wholly due to emphysema. This stems from a concern that morphine may make breathing worse rather than better in this group of people. Experience has not only shown this to be untrue but has also confirmed that morphine, if used correctly, eases the distress associated with breathlessness whether it is due to emphysema, heart failure or cancer.

Benzodiazepines

This class of drugs, of which valium is the best known, may be helpful in situations where breathlessness continues to be a problem despite the optimum use of morphine and oxygen. Small doses may be given during the day to ease distress and anxiety, with slightly larger doses at night to improve sleep. Sleep deprivation can be a major problem in those who are breathless and the benefits of a good night's sleep should not be underestimated.

Steroids

Steroids are occasionally helpful in treating breathlessness. By 'steroids' I do not mean those preparations used (illegally) by some athletes to build muscle but a special type of steroid that has an anti-inflammatory effect. This anti-inflammatory effect may help if breathlessness results from a cancer pressing on the airways or from lymphangitis. Lymphangitis is a relatively rare complication of cancer where the cancer spreads over the surface of the lung, limiting its capacity to expand. The steroids most commonly used are dexamethasone, prednisone and prednisolone. Benefits cannot be guaranteed but, when they do occur, they appear within days of starting treatment and may last for weeks to months. Steroids are occasionally tried but rarely help with other causes of breathlessness such as emphysema.

Radiotherapy

Radiotherapy has a very limited role in the treatment of breathlessness due to cancer. It is generally reserved for those whose cancer is pressing on one of the larger airways and whose life expectancy can be measured in months. The effect of radiotherapy is to shrink the cancer, allowing air to move more freely through the airway. Radiotherapy is generally not given when cancer is present within the substance of the lung even though this is a common cause of breathlessness. The normal lung is very sensitive to radiotherapy and the dose required to shrink the cancer may do more harm to the surrounding good lung.

What can you do for a severe episode of breathlessness?

◆ If oxygen is in the home but not in use, connect it up immediately and run it at maximum capacity (5 litres/ minute via a mask or nasal prongs for a concentrator; 8–10 litres/minute via a mask for a cylinder).

◆ If the oxygen is already attached, check that it is turned on and that there are no blockages in the system. Usually, there is a soft or loud whistling noise if a blockage is present. Make sure all the connections are firm. Then turn the flow rate to maximum capacity. If you are using a cylinder, ensure it is not empty.

◆ If you have both a cylinder and concentrator, use the cylinder in preference as you can run the oxygen at a higher flow rate.

◆ Sit your relative upright and open nearby windows.

◆ If your relative/friend has morphine as part of their regular medication, give a breakthrough dose.

◆ Ring the doctor and/or nurse as quickly as possible.

◆ Sit with the person until help arrives.

◆ With the help of your doctor, develop a plan to cope with possible future attacks.

Stridor

Stridor is the name given to a croup-like breathing that occasionally accompanies some malignancies in the chest. This whistling or high-pitched noise occurs when cancer (or lymphoma) presses on and narrows one of the larger airways (bronchus). The sound is heard during inspiration and expiration, and is usually present throughout waking and sleeping hours. It may be accompanied by a feeling of breathlessness and a dry unproductive cough. The combination of stridor and breathlessness can be distressing for the patient and you, the carer, and not uncommonly leads to a concern about suffocation. Suffocation is an extremely rare complication of cancer but, if you are worried about the possibility, discuss its prevention and treatment options with the doctor.

Cough

Cough is not a common complaint but is more likely to occur where cancer originates from or has spread to the lungs; it is also seen in those with emphysema or severe heart failure. With cancer, cough is often persistent and dry with little or no associated sputum. Occasionally, blood will be found in the sputum or it may seem as if blood is all that is being coughed up. The blood originates from the cancer, is bright red in colour and should be reported to the doctor. If coughing of blood is frequent or if the amount is considerable, radiotherapy is often recommended and can be very effective in stopping the bleeding. Coughing of blood also occurs in those with heart failure as a result of increasing congestion and is often treated with large doses of fluid tablets.

In the absence of blood, simple measures such as a cough mixture may be all that is required. If this fails and the cough is distressing, morphine in small doses is very effective in suppressing cough. Morphine is generally given by mouth but this is one of the few occasions when it may be more effective via a nebuliser and, if necessary, combined with other medications such as Ventolin. Occasionally, cough may be due to or aggravated by an underlying infection. If so, a course of antibiotics may help, but the relative merits of this form of treatment depend on the circumstances. Your doctor will assess the need and advise you on this matter.

Nausea and vomiting

Nausea and vomiting are two of the commonest symptoms associated with cancer and other life-threatening illnesses such as late-stage heart, liver and kidney disease. Both are very distressing symptoms, particularly in someone already weakened from the effects of serious illness. Nausea and vomiting are particularly common with cancer originating in the stomach or pancreas, or any cancer that has spread to the liver. If nausea and vomiting occur in association with cancer in other areas, or early in the course of an illness, a cause other than the cancer or illness should be sought.

There is a widely held belief that death follows quickly once cancer has spread to the liver. This is not altogether true, as the outcome depends more on the type of cancer and how fast it is growing than on the liver involvement itself. The liver is a remarkable organ and can continue to function for quite a long time even when much of it has been replaced by cancer. Some people have lived for many months, up to a year, despite liver involvement by cancer, whereas others have succumbed more quickly.

Causes (not in any order of frequency or importance) of nausea and vomiting other than cancer or the disease process include:

◆ constipation;

◆ blockage in the bowel;

◆ oral thrush or other mouth infections;

◆ kidney problems;

◆ excess calcium in the blood;

◆ medications including morphine, antibiotics, anti-inflammatory drugs, diuretics (fluid tablets) and some of the liquid preparations used to treat constipation;

◆ overfeeding—this commonly results from concerned

family members encouraging their relative to eat more than they want;

◆ a combination of any of the above.

The cause is often fairly clear-cut. If not, the doctor may suggest tests to look for or to exclude potentially reversible problems such as constipation. Constipation is one of the commonest and most overlooked causes of nausea and vomiting and must be considered before investigations and treatment are planned.

When medication is thought to be the cause, the offending drug(s) will probably be withdrawn and an equally effective alternative substituted. If the drug is essential and cannot be withdrawn, the addition of an antiemetic may be necessary. Overfeeding is not uncommon. It often involves a patient who has lost weight, and eating is encouraged in the mistaken belief that reversing the weight loss may reverse the downhill trend. Overfeeding, particularly if it induces vomiting, makes the situation worse rather than better (see section on weight loss in Chapter 5, Day-to-day care). Those with nausea and vomiting may not feel like eating but appetite may improve if a cause for the symptoms is found and treated. Until then it is best to let the person determine if and when they would like to eat, what type of food or liquid and in what quantity.

Nausea and vomiting caused by a cancer blocking the bowel is very difficult to treat. No amount of anti-vomiting medication is likely to eliminate the symptom entirely and surgery is generally not indicated in those with advanced cancer, not only because of their weakened state but also because the blockage is frequently not amenable to surgery. While medication may not stop the vomiting, it often reduces the frequency and is used for that reason. Please note: surgery may be considered in those not so sick or if this is their first episode of a bowel blockage.

With bowel obstruction, fluid intake is something that should be discussed with the doctor, but small amounts by mouth are usually recommended to ease thirst. Liquids taken by mouth are unlikely to make the vomiting worse, providing due care is taken with the type and volume of the fluids. Water and clear fluids like 'flat' lemonade are tolerated best. Intravenous or subcutaneous fluid replacement may or may not have a place.

Food intake is virtually a non-issue in people with a bowel blockage due to advanced cancer. They have little or no desire to eat and can barely tolerate the sight or smell of food. It is not uncommon in this situation for families to worry that not eating will result in death from starvation. Death in this setting is inevitable and does not result from lack of food (or fluid for that matter) but from the widespread effects of the cancer (see Chapter 5, Day-to-day care, for further information). Attempts at feeding in this situation are almost always counterproductive and further impair the quality of life.

Medication to improve nausea and vomiting

Numerous medications can be used to prevent or treat nausea and vomiting. These are called antiemetics. The most popular and commonly used antiemetics are as follows (generic name followed by brand name):

- haloperidol (Serenace)
- metoclopramide (Maxolon)
- domperidone (Motilium)
- prochlorperazine (Stemetil)
- promethazine (Phenergan)
- corticosteroids (Dexamethasone)
- ondansetron (Zofran)

Antiemetics are generally given by mouth except when vomiting is intractable. They are given then by injection under the skin to ensure adequate absorption. Depending on the cause, the doctor will usually start with one of the above drugs and will increase the dose, change the antiemetic or use a combination of them until the symptom has improved.

Antiemetic medication is prescribed to control and prevent vomiting so it is given regularly and continued even when the vomiting has settled. To withdraw treatment at that point may lead to a return of the symptom and that is something we all wish to avoid. Antiemetics are not free of side effects and may occasionally cause drowsiness or result in a restless-leg problem. Some aggravate Parkinson's disease and due caution must be exercised in choosing the appropriate drug in this situation.

Treatment of nausea and vomiting in end-stage heart, liver and kidney failure can be extremely difficult. The principles of treatment are much the same as with cancer—treatable causes are excluded and treated and antiemetics introduced when necessary. The nausea associated with kidney failure is often intractable but some of the newer antiemetics have proved more successful.

Difficulty with swallowing (dysphagia)

Dysphagia literally means pain with swallowing. If pain is the major problem, particularly if it is localised to the throat, thrush is a very likely cause. For further information, see under Mouth Care in Chapter 5, Day-to-day care. In the absence of thrush, difficulty with swallowing may be due to a blockage in the oesophagus, often but not always because of cancer. In this case, difficulty with swallowing is greatest with solid food rather than liquids; the person will often say food gets stuck and will indicate this by pointing to the lower neck or to the front of the chest.

If difficulty with swallowing is due to cancer, this inability to eat or drink is a turning point in the life of the person affected. Not only is it a serious complication but it puts the person and family in the difficult position of having to choose between invasive treatments and no treatment other than supportive care. This is as much a philosophical issue as a personal choice and whatever the decision, and irrespective of how it is made, there will often be questions and doubts along the way. Basically, the choice is between investigations followed by rather invasive treatment or a conservative approach that may involve subcutaneous fluids. The implications for life and death are clear. The resolution may not be so difficult if the person is clearly dying or if the symptom appears in someone who still has a good quality of life. The difficulty arises when there is uncertainty about prognosis. The decision will ultimately be based on the expressed wish of the person affected, after all possible options have been discussed.

In such an emotive situation it is not uncommon for there to be dissent within the family about the way to proceed—some will want active treatment while others may feel this is too cruel, given the circumstances. Consensus may or may not be achieved but it is important that everyone has the opportunity to express an opinion. Open discussion at this time, with the doctor and all family members present, can sometimes prevent long-term family rifts.

A full discussion of treatment options is beyond the scope of this book but possible interventions for swallowing difficulties due to cancer blocking the oesophagus include:

- radiotherapy;
- placement of a stent in the oesophagus to facilitate swallowing;
- insertion of a feeding or PEG tube to provide an alternative route for nutrition; the tube goes into the stomach via the abdominal wall and thus bypasses the blockage;
- intravenous or subcutaneous fluids.

For further information on any of these, speak to your doctor. If your loved one is not so well and a decision made not to intervene, treatment follows the course outlined under fluids in Chapter 5.

Loss of appetite

See Chapter 5, Day-to-day care.

Constipation

See Chapter 5, Day-to-day care.

Fatigue and weakness

Loss of appetite, loss of weight and loss of energy are very common accompaniments of cancer or any life-threatening illness and ultimately render people so weak they are unable to leave a chair or bed without assistance. The degree of weakness often (but not always) parallels the rate and degree of weight loss simply because of associated muscle wasting. You would think that giving a person good meals and protein supplements would reverse the problem or at least stop it in its tracks. Sadly, it doesn't. Loss of appetite is so marked that the person is unable to eat sufficient food to make a difference and, even if they could eat, their body is unable to process food in the usual way and much of the nutritional value is lost or utilised by the cancer. Many other factors such as inactivity, medication, depression, anaemia and metabolic problems contribute but are relatively minor players in the weakness.

According to many surveys, fatigue is one of the most distressing and disabling symptoms found in those who are dying. Unlike other troublesome symptoms such as pain, breathlessness, nausea and vomiting, there is little treatment that makes a difference. Not only does fatigue result in loss of independence, it also increases the risk of complications such as falls and pressure areas. The overall effect on quality of life is therefore quite significant.

Although there is no specific treatment, I offer a few suggestions on how best to help someone with weakness.

◆ Allow the person to do as little or as much as they want. Encouraging unrealistic activity in someone who is weak is not physically or psychologically helpful and may compromise safety.

◆ Loss of independence is the major consequence of weakness and both you and your loved one need to prepare for this by having the necessary equipment at home to help with the difficult tasks and to prevent accidents. An occupational therapist can advise on these matters.

◆ Safety and maintenance of dignity become increasingly important as weakness worsens.

◆ If you suspect depression is contributing to the inactivity, ask the doctor to assess the situation and advise on the relative merits of antidepressant medication, counselling and general supportive measures.

◆ Blood transfusion rarely makes a difference to weakness and fatigue in the later stages of illness and is inappropriate if death is near. If the person is not so ill, treatment of anaemia may be helpful if the physical deterioration corresponds with the onset of anaemia. In most cases, however, the overall benefits of transfusion in those with advanced disease is somewhat disappointing. Consider the matter carefully and discuss it fully with the doctor if anaemia is found to be present.

Hiccups

Although they are an infrequent complication of illness, hiccups may be troublesome and very difficult to palliate. They occur because of irritation to the diaphragm from cancer or because of a very full stomach when a bowel obstruction is present. In the latter case, careful attention to the quantity and frequency of fluid intake may improve the situation. The usual tricks, such as swallowing granulated sugar or holding one's breath, rarely work when hiccups occur in the presence of severe illness. These measures can be tried but, if the problem is ongoing and distressing, medication is often required. Again, there is no guarantee of success. Your doctor will advise you further about possible treatments but a drug called baclofen has proved to be successful when others have been tried and failed.

Ascites

Ascites is a swelling of the abdomen secondary to the accumulation of fluid within the abdominal cavity. It occurs commonly with certain cancers and advanced cirrhosis of the liver and occasionally with heart failure. The swelling may be very slight and not noticed by anyone other than the patient. They may be aware that underclothes are a little tighter round the waist or that belts need to be loosened. If the swelling increases, as it often does, the abdomen will become visibly distended and distinctly uncomfortable with the person complaining of fullness, bloating and discomfort. Breathing may be more difficult and in some cases the person is unable to lie flat. Often there is associated swelling of the ankles; sometimes, this can extend to or above the level of the knees.

The fluid generally accumulates freely within the abdominal cavity but occasionally it is confined to pockets. This distinction is only important if the fluid is to be drained and explains why your doctor may recommend an ultrasound before such a procedure. This investigation not only confirms the presence of ascites but also directs the doctor where to insert the drainage needle.

Drainage is a simple, painless and relatively safe procedure that can, if necessary, be performed in the person's home. A cannula (very similar to the cannula used for a drip) is inserted through the anaesthetised skin of the abdomen. The cannula is advanced until fluid begins to drain. A tube is then attached to the cannula and fluid runs through this system into a drainage bag. The volume that drains may be as small as 1 litre or as much as 10 litres. The duration of the procedure depends on the amount of fluid but rarely extends beyond a few hours. The person may sit in a chair or remain in bed while the fluid is draining.

Ascites is drained only if the associated symptoms warrant, and relief is then usually immediate. The fluid is rich in protein and the major drawback to the procedure is the loss of this valuable source of nutrition. For this reason, the procedure is only performed if symptoms warrant and not merely because fluid is present. The relief is unfortunately temporary as the fluid invariably reccumulates, often requiring further drainage within weeks or months. Drainage may aggravate pre-existing fatigue and weakness but this improves spontaneously within a few days and is helped by encouraging the person to drink fluids. Reducing the fluid intake does not prevent or reduce the rate at which fluid reaccumulates and will only make weakness and a dry mouth worse. Fluid tablets may be of some use if the ascites is due to liver or heart disease but are rarely of help with cancer.

Confusion or delirium

Confusion or, to be more exact, delirium is common in those dying of cancer, kidney failure or liver failure and the likelihood of it appearing increases as death approaches. Confusion manifests in numerous ways but most frequently as disturbed thinking, disorientation, seemingly unconnected thoughts and agitation. Behavioural accompaniments are common and often the earliest signs of a delirium. They may include inappropriate behaviour (e.g. looking at a book upside down or pouring tea onto breakfast cereal), wandering at night, insomnia and urinary incontinence.

The changes, although subtle, can be very distressing to behold. The delirious person often has some insight into their problem and may have periods of lucidity when they feel embarrassed about what they have done or the inconvenience they have caused. Your gentle messages of love and understanding will go a long way towards comforting and reassuring them as well as settling the delirium, albeit temporarily.

While delirium may be an inevitable accompaniment of illness and dying, the reason for its appearance is complex and often related to a combination of factors. In the context of cancer, however, two questions invariably arise: Is the delirium due to morphine? Has the cancer spread to the brain?

Is the delirium a result of morphine?

Morphine may cause or contribute to delirium and the likelihood increases as the dose increases. So, delirium from morphine should be considered when a large dose is currently in use or when the onset of delirium is closely related to the commencement of morphine or to an increase in its dose. As delirium caused by morphine is almost always dose-related, an appropriate reduction in the dose often improves the situation without compromising pain relief. Reductions are made slowly and incrementally becasue a more rapid reduction in dosage could result in a flare-up of pain. This is not only distressing but can also make the confusion worse. If the delirium is marked and morphine thought to be the likely cause, the doctor may choose to cease morphine altogether and substitute an equally effective analgesic. I would not like to leave you with the idea that morphine is the commonest cause of delirium in someone with cancer. It may be the first cause your doctor thinks of, but only because it is the easiest to treat.

The likelihood of delirium increases as death approaches, and the complications and physiological changes associated with this deterioration is what predisposes to the delirium. Such changes include an altered metabolism, kidney and liver problems, and some forms of infection. Given better circumstances, these may be amenable to treatment but, in someone who is dying, the burden of change is so great as to render treatment virtually ineffective. This situation is akin to putting out spot fires while a bush fire rages out of control all around.

Treatment aimed at reversing these problems when a person is dying is therefore futile, can add to discomfort and may do more harm than good. When death is inevitable it is better to concentrate all efforts on making death and what remains of life as dignified as possible. This does not automatically exclude a search for a cause, but the proximity to death rather than the degree of confusion will determine how appropriate this may be.

Has the cancer spread to the brain?

Contrary to popular belief, a 'brain' tumour is a relatively uncommon cause of delirium, irrespective of whether it has arisen in or spread to the brain. Brain tumours may sometimes cause delirium but it is not an automatic association. In other words, if a person with a brain tumour becomes confused other causes need to be considered before the confusion is attributed to the tumour. How actively this line of investigation is pursued (if at all) will depend on the overall state of the person concerned more than the degree of confusion. If the person is unwell and close to death, investigation is unlikely to alter the outcome and efforts aimed at maintaining comfort and dignity will ultimately be more beneficial. The outcome may be more beneficial in those who are less sick, as Isabel's case illustrates.

Isabel was in her early sixties and had a very rapidly growing cancer that had spread to her bones. She was depressed and had quite a lot of pain that ultimately improved with morphine. Over four to eight weeks her husband had noticed minor but uncharacteristic changes in her behaviour and thought patterns. He was prompted to report these only after Isabel attempted to get out of a moving car. Examination and tests revealed no obvious cause for the delirium and the situation did not improve after the morphine dose was reduced. A brain scan did not show a definite tumour although there were some changes that suggested the cancer may have spread to the surface of the brain.

Isabel was admitted to the local hospice with a view to investigating the problem further, to commence treatment and manage her potentially dangerous behaviour. As is customary, all medication that seemed unnecessary was ceased at the time of admission. Within days there was a small but significant improvement in Isabel's mental state and after one week she was virtually back to normal. A review of the medication led us to conclude the delirium was due to an antidepressant that had been started just before the delirium was first noted. Subsequent review of the medical literature confirmed this drug does indeed cause delirium.

People with cancer are more susceptible to the side effects of most medications. So if delirium should occur, ask the doctor to review the treatment and, if possible, reduce the dose of those that must be continued and stop those that are no longer necessary.

What can you do to improve delirium?

◆ If the person is confused about time and place, orientate them as often as necessary by telling them where they are and what is happening.

◆ If there is one thing that appears to be troubling your relative, listen and allow them to tell the full story. A friend of mine who is dying has recently become confused. She asks where she is and where is her bed. When I remind her she is in her bed and in her home, this always has a marked settling effect. As a result, I now introduce myself when I visit, tell her the time of day and the day of the week. I take nothing for granted. I explain what I am doing or about to do (e.g. feed her), tell her about any noise that may be audible (e.g. washing machine, outside traffic) and let her know who is in the house when I leave. This seems to orientate her and help minimise the confusion.

◆ Keep familiar photos and favourite objects nearby.

◆ Keep the environment as constant as possible. Sensory overload with lots of different visitors or frequent changes of scenery can add to the confusion.

◆ Be aware of safety issues—for example, do not leave dangerous items nearby, supervise the drinking of hot fluids, take care with heaters.

◆ Delirium is often worse at night—familiar background music and a soft night-light may help.

◆ If the delirium is marked, a roster may need to be drawn up to ensure a familiar face is always present.

◆ If all these measures have been tried and delirium is persistent, distressing, undignified or potentially dangerous, medication may be required. There are several treatment options and your doctor will discuss them if or when it becomes necessary.

Fitting

Fitting is an uncommon complication of cancer and is even less frequent with other life-threatening illnesses. Fitting is distressing for all concerned and often provokes anxiety in the carer who, faced with a potential crisis, may be frightened and uncertain how best to respond.

The most common form of fit is called a 'grand mal'. In this the person's body initially stiffens and this is followed by jerking movements (fitting) that involve the whole body but are most obvious in the arms and legs. The fit may be as short as a few seconds or as long as several minutes; during this time, breathing is noisy, skin colour changes from pink to a bluish hue and there may be incontinence of urine and faeces. The person is unconscious throughout the fit and for some time after, and will therefore have no recollection of the event. When the fitting stops, as it invariably does, the person may sleep for a short time and breathing and colour will gradually return to normal. A brief period of confusion is not uncommon after they 'come to' and during this time it is important to reassure them, as they are often vaguely aware that something has happened.

With the full blown or grand mal fit the following measures are recommended.

- Do not attempt to restrain the person while they are twitching as this may result in bruising and injury.

- Do not attempt to put a peg or other object between the teeth. Apart from being a near impossible task, it does no good and may break teeth or dislodge dentures.

- If they are in bed, ensure as best you can they do not fall to the floor. If they are on the floor, leave them as you find them but use pillows or blankets to prevent their head, arms or legs hitting against fixed objects.

- If the person does not regain consciousness immediately after the fitting has ceased, lay them on their side and remove any dentures.

- Commence oxygen after the fit has stopped or earlier if the fit is prolonged. This is not essential so do not be alarmed if you do not have oxygen.

- Notify a doctor or nurse and then sit by the person until help arrives.

- It is not necessary to ring an ambulance unless a second fit occurs and only then if the doctor is unable to come immediately.

- When the person wakes tell them what has happened but reassure them that everything is under control. This is particularly important if the person is confused.

- Confusion is almost certainly a result of the fit and should settle within minutes or hours.

Sometimes the fit may be partial with the jerking movements confined to one side of the body or parts thereof. There is no loss of consciousness with this type of fit, and colour and breathing remain unchanged. Reassurance is particularly important in this instance, as the person is fully aware of what is happening, is likely to be frightened and may even wonder if they are about to die. Again, the doctor or palliative care nurse should be notified.

Whether the fit is full blown or partial the doctor will almost certainly prescribe medication to prevent further fits. This is usually in tablet or capsule form but an injection may be given in the first instance. Depending on the state of health of the person and the anticipated life expectancy, investigations may be done to determine the cause of the fit.

Fits are not an invariable consequence of brain tumours—in fact, they are relatively uncommon. For this reason medication to prevent fits is rarely given when a brain tumour is diagnosed unless there has been a previous fit. There are a few exceptions. Some tumours are more likely to cause fits if they spread to the brain and it is not unusual for anticonvulsant medication to be given prophylactically in these situations. If your relative/friend has a 'tumour' that involves the brain, you can ask the doctor about the need for tablets to prevent fits or injections to be kept in the home in case a fit should occur.

Ankle swelling

Oedema, or swelling of the ankles and legs, occurs in those with heart, liver or kidney failure and will appear at some stage in the course of cancer. In the later stages of cancer the swelling is often secondary to weight loss or other nutritional changes that are common around this time. Blood clots (deep vein thrombosis) are relatively common in those who are sick, particularly if they are confined to bed or a chair, and may at times be responsible for swelling. Whatever the cause, protein-rich water accumulates under the skin and causes swelling. It is first seen in the ankle region, gradually extends upwards and may involve the whole of both legs and lower trunk. Pain does not normally accompany the swelling but the legs may be tender to touch. If pain is present, a blood clot is possible and this may require specific treatment. Depending on the amount of swelling, heaviness of the legs may also be a problem. Water is heavy and the added weight can make it difficult for the person to lift their legs. It can limit activity, compromise independence and introduce safety issues.

The skin over the swelling is often tissue paper thin and can tear with the slightest trauma. These tears may be microscopic or large and allow the fluid to seep out, resulting in dampness of clothing and bed linen. If this occurs, the legs should be bandaged to contain the seepage and also to protect against further skin damage. The protein-rich fluid is a favourite culture medium for many bugs and so due care must be taken to prevent infection whenever a tear is present.

Elevating the legs helps to redistribute the fluid to other parts of the body and explains why ankle swelling improves after a night in bed and is worse after prolonged sitting or standing. For this reason it is helpful to keep the legs elevated when the person is sitting, but don't insist if it is too uncomfortable. Massage can also redistribute the fluid but is not something I recommend, bearing in mind the delicate nature of the skin and the possibility of tears. The gentle application of sorbolene cream to the affected areas, particularly if the skin is dry, may reduce the likelihood of tears by helping to preserve skin integrity.

Elastic stockings may help to reduce swelling in those who are up and about or who spend much of their day in a chair. The benefits are marginal and the nuisance value high. Stockings may be hot in summer, uncomfortable and/or unbecoming and so the potential benefits need to be weighed against these disadvantages. Fluid tablets are occasionally used to reduce swelling but their success rate is low and the incidence of side effects high. For this reason they are reserved for the 'relatively well' and even in that group great care must to be taken in the choice and dose of medication. Their use is inappropriate and dangerous in those who are less well and completely out of place in those who are close to death.

Sweating

Sweating can be a troublesome symptom in anyone who is unwell. It occurs frequently and may be caused by infection, a side effect of medication (morphine and paracetamol are the main offenders) or the illness itself (particularly lymphoma, leukaemia and widespread cancer). The sweats are more likely to occur at night, are frequently drenching and often require a change of night attire and bed linen. Treatment involves looking for and treating any cause (if appropriate) as well as the following comfort measures.

◆ Ensure the room is not too hot.

◆ Open windows or use a fan to circulate the air.

◆ Avoid warm clothing and too many blankets.

◆ Cotton clothing and bed linen are less likely to induce sweating than those made of synthetic fibres.

◆ Change pyjamas and bed linen as required.

◆ Encourage the person to drink ample fluids.

In cases where the sweating is profuse and the above measures fail to offer relief, several medications have been trialled with varying degrees of success. Your doctor can tell you more about the relative merits of such treatment.

Infections

Chest infections are particularly common in those with cancer of the lung, a history of chest troubles such as emphysema and those confined to bed. The infection generally manifests in the usual way with a moist cough and coloured sputum but, occasionally, these signs are absent and the only tell-tale sign may be a sudden deterioration in the person's health.

Other sites of possible infection include the skin, bladder, kidney and blood. Skin infections or abscesses may occur around a pressure area or at the site of a previous injection or butterfly needle. Bladder and kidney infections are more common in those with urinary catheters or cancer in the pelvic region (e.g. prostate cancer in men and cervical, uterine or ovarian cancer in women). Blood infection (septicaemia) is generally seen in the very sick, those with leukaemia or lymphoma and those who are jaundiced. As with pneumonia, septicaemia can lead to a sudden and dramatic deterioration.

In those not so unwell, infections are nearly always treated with an appropriate antibiotic. Depending on the site of the infection, other specific measures may also be necessary. For example, a skin abscess may need to be lanced, a butterfly needle changed if the surrounding skin is swollen and a urinary catheter removed or replaced if it is thought to be the cause of a kidney infection.

The use of antibiotics in someone close to death is a difficult and complex matter as antibiotics at this time may be futile and inappropriate. I do not wish to imply that antibiotic treatment should never be given to someone who is dying; the decision should be weighed carefully and guided by the known or expressed wish of that person as well as their state of health.

Itch

Itch is not a common problem but is mentioned because of the distress it can cause. It is often present in those with jaundice and is at its worst when the jaundice is due to a blockage to the flow of bile, as occurs with cancer of the pancreas or cancer of the biliary tree. The deeper the jaundice the worse the itch. At times the itch may be so bad as to interfere with sleep and cause marked restlessness throughout the day. Itch may also result from the use of morphine and may appear as part of an allergic reaction to certain drugs, particularly antibiotics. An alternative pain reliever to morphine or a change of antibiotics resolves these problems. Itch is also relatively common with some lymphomas.

When there is no obvious or treatable cause, some improvement may result from the use of antihistamine tablets or skin preparations such as calamine lotion. Night sedation may help to overcome any associated sleep disturbance but it is not uncommon to see people scratching even during sleep. If the skin is damaged or bleeds because of the intense scratching, mittens may be helpful at night. Heat can also make the itch worse.

Relief of itch associated with jaundice comes only from relieving the jaundice. This may or may not be possible and depends on the state of the person and the extent of the cancer. In those not so sick, the blockage to the flow of bile may be relieved surgically or by means of a semi-rigid tube (stent) that can be inserted through and beyond the obstruction, permitting the normal flow of bile to resume thereby relieving the jaundice. This is much simpler and less risky than surgery but has the disadvantage of providing only temporary relief. A stent may be removed and a new one reinserted but each successive procedure becomes more difficult and ultimately impossible. Stents are prone to infection but respond to appropriate antibiotic treatment. Surgery gives a longer lasting result but is often too dangerous a proposition for those with advanced cancer.

A drug called cholestyramine is sometimes used when itch is due to jaundice and cannot be palliated by surgery or stenting. It comes as powder and needs to be taken three or four times a day. It has an unpleasant taste, is constipating and rarely results in anything more than a slight improvement— not much of a recommendation!

Haemorrhage

Loss of blood may occur internally (and is therefore not visible) or through any orifice, when it may appear with vomiting, coughing, in a bowel motion, while urinating or spontaneously through the vagina. The amount can be small or quite substantial and is then associated with pallor and sweating. Haemorrhage should always be reported to your doctor or nurse and the degree of urgency will depend on the volume lost and the physical and emotional state of your loved one. The loss of smaller amounts of blood (streaks or spots) is much less significant but should be reported as a matter of routine, though not urgently.

The possibility of haemorrhage should be discussed with the doctor and, if there is more than a remote chance of it occurring, a plan of action should be drawn up. See the end of this chapter for more information.

Insomnia

Difficulty with sleeping is not unusual for someone who is ill or dying. Pain, bodily discomfort, difficulty with breathing and other symptoms are not conducive to a good night's sleep. Inactivity, a different bed and an unfamiliar environment may also play a part. Fear of dying in one's sleep, fear of the future and existential crises are frequent and often overlooked causes. Irrespective of the cause(s) a long sleepless night has a deleterious effect on the healthy, so imagine what it must be like for someone who is unwell.

Physical and emotional problems always seem worse when we are alone and a night without sleep can magnify them even more. For those who are dying, a sleepless night may open a Pandora's box of thoughts and emotions. The loneliness of dying, the sadness of leaving those they love, uncertainty about the future, the fear of suffering, the fear that death may come that night and bodily pain all loom large and become more sinister in the long dark hours of the night. It is no wonder those who are ill dread the night and often have difficulty sleeping.

While all this may sound bad, it can also be seen as an opportunity for healing. This may seem odd—how can something so emotionally traumatic benefit anyone, particularly someone who is dying? The following example may help to illustrate the point.

Barbara had been admitted to the hospice because of pain from widespread cancer. She was in her early forties, happily married with one teenage daughter. According to her family, she had until that time managed reasonably well at home, showing few signs of emotional distress. She had the occasional episode of panic, often while in the bathroom, but only when the door was shut. She had overcome this quite simply by leaving the bathroom door open.

Pain medication was adjusted and after several days Barbara had little if any daytime pain and was seen to be fairly active around the ward. The nights were a different story. She was unable to sleep 'because of pain' and asked for regular breakthrough doses of morphine. According to the night staff, this resulted in short periods of sleep but pain was always present when she woke 1–2 hours later.

The night staff was very astute and felt there was more behind the wakefulness than pain and decided to spend time with her when she woke at night. During these times Barbara slowly opened up and spoke of her anxiety about what was happening, her fear of dying, her concern for her family and how she was unlikely now to do many of the things she had always wanted to do. During these outpourings Barbara did not once complain of pain and more often than not would go to sleep without the assistance of pain medication or sedation. After several nights of talking and expression of emotions Barbara became more settled, required no extra pain medication and slept for long periods throughout the night.

While the night may bring darkness it somewhat paradoxically puts the spotlight on all the fears and concerns that have been neatly tucked away. Daytime activities are very effective in keeping emotions out of sight and out of mind but the stillness of the night often sees them well up and catch us by surprise. In Barbara's case the worsening pain carried a strong message that the cancer was getting worse.

This raised many fears and concerns which she managed to keep at bay while at home even though the panic episodes suggested they were very close to the surface.

 Anxiety is a better teacher than reality, for reality can be temporarily avoided whereas anxiety is ever present.

SOREN KIERKEGAARD

In the unfamiliar hospice situation, with no husband to comfort her at night, Barbara was helpless to fend off the emotions that welled up during those long dark hours. What she called 'pain' was not physical pain but suffering and, not surprisingly, morphine did little to help. The brief periods of sleep simply put everything on hold until she woke, and when she did the 'demons' were still there. Desmond Tutu, in his book *No Future Without Forgiveness*, says 'unless you look the beast in the eye you will find that it returns to hold you hostage'.

Talking about fears and concerns is one way of confronting the beasts and, in the case of insomnia, is often a more fruitful way of dealing with the problem than resorting to sedation or 'pain' relief. At times, sedation may indeed be useful and necessary but care must be taken to ensure the cause of the insomnia is always addressed. Sometimes it is pain or another physical problem but, as with Barbara, there may be a deeper cause.

If the problem is physical pain or some other symptom, attending to that will improve sleep. It may be that inactivity and frequent daytime dozes make sleep at night harder to come by. If so, a change to the daily routine may be a more satisfactory alternative to sedation. If there are clear signs of emotional distress, allowing the person to talk will be an important part of the care and healing.

Sedation has a limited role but may be used for brief

periods to re-establish a normal sleep pattern if this has been disturbed by hospitalisation or an altered home environment.

If night sedation is used, do remember:

◆ Morning drowsiness is a potential problem particularly if sedation is given later than the recommended time.

◆ The risk of a fall or other accident increases with the degree of drowsiness.

◆ The elderly and frail are more at risk of excessive sedation and so the dose may need to be adjusted in these groups.

◆ A previous history of sedative or heavy alcohol use or drug abuse may render the prescribed sedation less effective.

◆ Sedation loses its effect over time so is best used for brief periods only.

◆ Sedation may occasionally cause or contribute to the onset of confusion.

◆ If reasonable doses of sedation do not achieve the desired effect, consider underlying emotional or physical problems and address them if found.

How do I deal with emergencies?

The likelihood of an emergency is generally small but being prepared helps you to be forearmed. The most frequently encountered emergencies are listed below. This book provides basic information on most of them but the finer details need to be worked out with the treating doctor. So sit down with the doctor, discuss what crises, if any, may occur and what you should do at those times. In other words, formulate a plan. Every situation is different and the way that you and the doctor plan to deal with an emergency will depend on circumstances and geography as well as on the underlying illness. Once the plan has been made, document it and make sure it is kept in a prominent place and that all key people know about it. Ensure you have all the medication and equipment that may be required. Check that you have the phone numbers of the people you may need to call. Record business, after-hour and mobile phone numbers and keep these in a very visible spot (e.g. the fridge door or by the phone).

Emergencies that may require forward planning include:

◆ sudden or severe pain;

◆ severe breathlessness;

◆ sudden loss of consciousness;

◆ sudden death;

◆ fitting;

◆ haemorrhage (bleeding);

◆ marked confusion;

◆ blocked urinary catheter;

◆ profuse or persistent vomiting;

◆ falls and/or fractures.

5 Day-to-day care

... the pauses between the notes—ah there is where the artistry lies.

ARTUR SACHNABEL

*t*his chapter deals with many of the practical problems encountered in the daily care of a person who is dying. It does not delve into medical or treatment-related issues, as these are covered in other chapters. Instead, it focuses on the basic necessities of life such as food, drink and comfort and how these are provided at the various stages of illness, particularly around the time of death (in palliative circles this form of care is called *supportive care*). Finally, it looks at the quality of human contact and how best to nurture and preserve the dignity of the person who is dying. The comments and observations are made with cancer in mind but most apply in varying degrees to other life-threatening illnesses.

The importance of supportive care hardly needs to be emphasised. From the moment your loved one receives a life-threatening diagnosis, you will expend extraordinary amounts of time and energy attempting to nurture their body as well as their spirit. When treatment fails and is ultimately withdrawn these basic human necessities assume even greater significance, as they alone are seen to stand between life and death. Food and fluids, once consumed for sustenance and pleasure, now take on alchemical proportions as, together with comfort measures, they become nature's medicine in the face of death.

The value attached to food and fluids can vary enormously within families, and these differences can cause problems. Some see the dwindling intake as part of the dying process and, while saddened, they accept the inevitability of death. Others are not so prepared to make the shift and may insist on special diets, vitamins or some form of artificial feeding in the belief that these will relieve suffering and change the course of events. If differences exist within the family of the one who is dying, repercussions may be considerable and long-lasting unless resolved early in the course of events.

If the dying person has given some form of care directive, all management decisions should flow according to that directive. If no such directive exists and the dying person does not or cannot express their wish, a family conference with the treating doctor present may resolve the impasse. In most instances, family differences, whether over food, fluids or whatever, can be bridged through good communication. An honest appraisal of the medical and emotional state of the dying person as well as the relative merits of the various treatments will assist in the process. This type of information, given compassionately and clearly, usually forms the basis of a successful resolution.

The need to feed someone who is clearly dying often arises from deep-seated grief. This grief is not helped by mis-information about the value of food or misconceptions about the level of suffering associated with not eating or drinking. The information that follows should go some way to clearing up misconceptions about food, fluids and other forms of supportive care.

Cancer cures

When someone is told they have cancer, they and their family go in search of treatments that may increase the chance of survival. This is a normal and healthy response but can sometimes get out of hand, consuming the life and time of many people in the process. The treatments I am referring to fall into two categories, medical and complementary.

Considerable uncertainty may exist about the value of medical treatment, particularly chemotherapy and radio-therapy. The benefits they offer are often accompanied by side effects that are unpleasant as well as unwanted. Despite this, most people with cancer will endure the physical and psychological blows associated with either or both of these treatments in the hope that the end result will justify the means. Their life may become an endless series of doctor's appointments, clinic visits, tests and predictions, but they subject themselves to these treatments that ravage the body and dislocate the soul in the hope of preserving life.

The situation with complementary (alternative) therapies is not much different. The range of complementary therapies on offer is enormous and increasing at a rapid rate. People will try almost anything. Many with cancer will, at some stage of their illness, experiment with a form of complementary therapy and evidence suggests that more money is spent on this treatment than on all the chemotherapy combined. When there is so much at stake, who can blame a person for trying? From the patient's point of view there is much to gain and nothing to lose, even if the medical profession sees it differently.

Diets, vitamin supplements and purported cancer cures have had little if any impact on the outcome of cancer. We could say much the same of chemotherapy, although there have been some spectacular remissions and cures with it. We must be careful not to judge those who go in search of cures but try to understand why they do it. People seek these treatments just as they seek chemotherapy, not as a last-ditch measure but as an opportunity to take some control over their destiny, rather than submit passively to an illness that threatens their existence. It becomes a visible and tangible way of expressing their desire to live.

If the treatments fail, we must avoid automatically labelling them as 'failures' and the person's efforts in vain. The example of Judy in Chapter 9, The inner journey, shows that any treatment, medical or complementary, cannot be judged only on whether it is successful but on what it has meant to the person and how it has influenced their life's journey. I am supportive of most complementary therapies providing:

- it has been a considered decision and not a reaction to something heard about from friends, relatives or the media;
- it is what the dying person wants rather than what a family member or friend recommends;
- it is done at an appropriate time in the illness and not at the eleventh hour;
- it does not consume too much valuable time or involve unreasonable travel;
- it is within the budget;
- it is not unpleasant, dangerous or clearly fraudulent;
- it does not interfere with standard treatments;
- it does not involve too great a change to the way of life or interfere with pleasurable activities, including the consumption of favourite foods or drinks;
- a time is set down to review the treatment and decide whether it will be continued.

Loss of appetite

Loss of appetite (anorexia) is one of the commonest complaints in those with cancer. The associated weight loss is not only the visible manifestation of this symptom but also a stark reminder of the illness and its devastating effects. While your first reaction will be to believe that the loss of appetite and/or weight loss is due to the cancer (or other illness), and may therefore be an ominous sign, it should be remembered there are many other possible causes. The list is long but chemotherapy, radiotherapy and other medications deserve special mention. More will be said about these and other causes of poor appetite later in this chapter.

When the anorexia is due to cancer, the rate and degree of weight loss closely reflects the state of the cancer. Unfortunately, the reverse is not always true—that is, the absence of weight loss or its temporary reversal does not automatically mean the cancer is static or improving.

If treatable causes have been excluded, numerous medical and proprietary lines are available that may stimulate appetite. Unfortunately, most have no measurable effect; of those that do, the benefit is usually short-lived or side effects preclude their long-term use. Your doctor is in the best position to advise you on what is available and can monitor the effects of treatment if you decide to proceed. The most frequently prescribed appetite stimulants are cortisone derivatives (usually dexamethasone) or a hormonal agent called megestrol. Cortisone is the more popular, but like megestrol its success rate is disappointingly low and benefits are temporary.

Weight loss

The body is like any machine and needs fuel to operate. This fuel comes in the form of food and fluids, which supply calories for the body to burn just as a motor car burns petrol. The number of calories we need each day to maintain normal function depends on our age, metabolism and level of activity. What may be sufficient for an elderly, inactive individual would be grossly inadequate for an active teenager in the middle of a growth spurt.

If we exceed our daily caloric needs we put on weight and if this continues unabated we risk becoming obese. If our caloric intake is inadequate we lose weight. Starvation is the extreme form of weight loss, seen in previous years in prisoners of war and today in adults and children in war-torn or developing countries. Anorexia nervosa is perhaps the closest thing to starvation that we see in our contemporary western world.

Like the motor car, the body has its own fuel tank where energy is stored for use when required. If fuel (calories) is in short supply and the level in the tank drops, the body adapts by slowing its metabolism, thereby reducing the need for fuel. If this is inadequate and the fuel tank runs dry, energy is obtained from fat stores, which act as a reserve tank. If the shortage continues for a prolonged period, body fat and then muscle will gradually disappear, the person becomes thinner and weaker and ultimately wasted, a condition we call cachexia. This sequence of changes is characteristic of starvation but not cancer.

When weight loss is due to inadequate intake of calories, as with starvation, replacing the calories, either naturally with food or artificially with intravenous or other forms of feeding, provides an immediate source of energy for the body to heal itself. Weight loss ceases, fat stores are replenished, physical strength returns, the fuel tank is topped up and the person looks and feels better.

Most people assume that all forms of weight loss result from inadequate food/calorie intake but this is not altogether true for cancer. Poor appetite and weight loss may be due to any number of causes—medication, chemotherapy, radiotherapy, surgery, difficulty with swallowing, peptic ulcers or other intercurrent illnesses. These causes are more common in the early stages of illness and, if present, appropriate treatment may improve appetite and reverse weight loss. As cancer advances and potentially toxic chemotherapy is withdrawn, loss of weight is nearly always related to the disease itself.

When weight loss occurs because of starvation the body attempts to minimise the loss by slowing the metabolic rate. With cancer the metabolic rate is high and remains high even when food intake is diminished or altogether absent. The reason for this aberration is complex but may be simplified as follows. Cancer is essentially a parasite, living on and deriving energy from its host (the patient), and it continues to grow irrespective of how much or how little the person eats. It is unresponsive to the mechanisms that control normal body functions. Even when there is a shortage of calories, cancer cells continue to grow and derive energy from their host, who loses weight. The greater the number of cancer cells (i.e. the bigger the cancer), the bigger the problem. It is this self-perpetuating parasitic action that keeps the metabolic rate high and results in rapid and dramatic weight loss (see Table 5.1).

Giving food to those whose weight loss is due to starvation quickly and effectively reverses the problem. Unfortunately, the same is not true of cancer. Food will not reverse the weight loss because it feeds the cancer as much as it provides nourishment for the body. Because its metabolic rate is so high the cancer soaks up the greater part of the calories while normal tissues miss out. This does not mean you should withhold food from someone with cancer, but food should be given only when desired. Feeding someone who has advanced cancer when they are not hungry does not make them feel better nor does it result in any increase in weight. The same principles apply to anyone with a life-threatening illness.

Loss of appetite with cancer makes some sense and can be seen as the body's way (futile as it may be) of dealing with the problem. It is as if the body recognises its dilemma and switches off its appetite in a desperate attempt to rid itself of the cancer.

TABLE 5.1 Changes associated with loss of weight due to starvation and cancer

	STARVATION	CANCER
Sensation of hunger	Yes (in early stages)	No
Metabolic rate	Decreased	Increased
Energy source	Fat	Fat and muscle
Effect of eating	Reverses weight loss	Weight loss continues
Effect of IV feeding	Beneficial	Counterproductive

All this has implications for cancer patients and the way their weight loss is treated. Similarly, the decision for or against intravenous or other artificial means of feeding depends very much on the cause of the problem. The closer someone is to death the more likely the poor appetite and weight loss is due to the cancer itself and not some other cause. It is therefore unlikely to respond to any form of intervention.

Food

Most but not all who are dying, particularly those with cancer, will lose their appetite at some stage. A time will come when the very sight or smell of food may induce nausea. When this happens, it is best to let the dying person dictate what and when they wish to eat and in what amounts. This is often harder than it sounds as the preparation and presentation of food may be one of the few remaining ways you can demonstrate your love and be of practical help. Meals and meal times are more than occasions to eat. They are times of sharing. They are part of the fabric of life. Dispensing with these established routines and traditions can be very painful. Your loved one's dying involves letting go of many things and, for some, food will be one of the losses.

 We so desperately want everything to continue as it is. Learning to live is learning to let go.
SOGYAL RIMPOCHE, *The Tibetan Book of Living and Dying*

Diets of any form (including that for diabetes), health foods and vitamin supplements have by this time outlived their usefulness and should be abandoned unless your relative/friend determines otherwise. Hanging on to these vestiges of treatment often says more about emotional than medical needs and that may need to be addressed more than the weight loss.

The ritual of three meals a day, while natural for the healthy, is totally inappropriate for those with advanced cancer or any life-threatening illness. Feeding should be determined by the wishes of the person, not the time of day. Servings should be small and presented on small plates, as the sight of a large amount of food can destroy whatever appetite remains. Allow the person to feed themselves if this is possible. They value this independence and it gives them control over how much food they want and how slowly they wish to eat it. It may upset you to see how little they consume, but don't be tempted to suggest they eat a little more. If you say this or attempt to feed them more, they may take it, not because they want it but to please you. Remember, their appetite is almost non-existent and what appears a mere morsel to you may be more than enough to satisfy their wants.

Angela was an elderly woman dying of cancer, being cared for by a loving extended family in her own home. Vomiting had been a major ongoing problem for which no cause could be found and all medications had been ineffective in relieving the problem. During one of my visits I noticed Angela was being fed a large meal that would have satisfied the heartiest of appetites. Angela's appetite was almost non-existent but she ate to please her family who believed feeding was essential for her well-being.

When asked, Angela said her appetite had all but gone and the very sight of food often made her sick. Hearing this, the family agreed to give her what she wanted and only when she wanted it. The vomiting all but stopped and, although her health continued to deteriorate, everyone was grateful this most distressing symptom had settled.

Certain foods seem to be more popular than others. Ice cream, yoghurt, custard, jelly (in fact, most sweets), smoothies, soups and small sandwiches (without the crust) are frequently eaten while 'mains' are left untouched. Tastes do differ, so don't take my word—ask your relative/friend what they would like and make sure you have ample supplies of their preferred food. Given the situation, the various nutritional supplements available through chemist shops have no advantage over smoothies or their like.

Thirst is often a greater concern than hunger so do not be surprised if the desire for fluid outweighs the desire for food. The rule of thumb is to give whatever fluids the person wants, in the amount they choose. Chilled or iced water is the most refreshing but soft drinks, cordials and fruit drinks are frequently requested and provide some variety. Small amounts of alcohol are permitted.

As the illness progresses, the dying person becomes increasingly weak and swallowing more of an ordeal. Appetite has by this time all but disappeared. When your loved one is unable to swallow or if they refuse food, concentrate on overall comfort. This includes keeping the mouth moist with small amounts of fluid or ice to suck (further information follows). Be reassured your relative or friend will not feel hungry and will not die of hunger. They are dying as a result of the illness, and the inability to eat and drink at this late stage is part of the dying process. Do not be side-tracked into doing something about their eating when it is their dying that demands your full attention. They need you much more than they need food.

Just as there is no place for food at this stage of a person's life there is also no role for intravenous fluids. Intravenous fluids have negligible nutritional value and do not make the dying person feel better; nor do they result in them living longer. Intravenous fluids may in fact make things worse. (I say more about this below.)

It is okay for you to drink or chew on something small while in the room but save larger meals for some other time and place. The sight and smell of your food may not be the best thing for someone already nauseated. If, on the other hand, the person asks you to sit and eat your meal with them, do so as this may indicate a desire to talk.

Fluids

While hunger is rarely a problem in those who are dying, the same cannot be said of thirst. The desire for liquids to quench thirst or soothe a parched throat is a constant problem. Thirst rarely influences the timing of death but it can certainly impair quality of life and cause physical discomfort around the time of death. The relief of thirst is one of the body's most basic needs and is present throughout life, from birth to death. Fluids are so vital to life that the body has many in-built warning devices to let it know if 'fluid levels' are too low. Thirst happens to be one of the very early warning signals. Initially, its message is gentle but if it goes unheard thirst increases and can become distinctly unpleasant. The most common causes of thirst are as follows.

◆ *Inadequate fluid intake.* This is the most obvious and frequently the most common cause of thirst. The average daily requirement for a healthy person is 1500–2000 ml/day (equivalent to 6–8 cups). Illness may render a person less active but their fluid requirement remains unchanged and is no different from that of a healthy person. Keeping up with this intake can be difficult, particularly if the person depends on others for help.

◆ *Increased fluid requirements.* Fluid requirements may be greater than normal because of any or all of the following:
 —adverse environmental conditions (e.g. a hot day);
 —sweating—a relatively common problem in those with advanced cancer, resulting in quite marked fluid loss;
 —fever and infection;
 —vomiting, diarrhoea or fluid loss from any cause;
 —medications—for example, fluid tablets (diuretics).

◆ *Dry mouth.* Causes include:
 —mouth infections, particularly thrush;

—morphine and other pain relievers, irrespective of whether they are given by mouth, injection or via a nebuliser;

—oxygen, either by mask or nasal prongs; it can dry the mouth and nasal passages when given without a humidifier.

When trying to prevent or alleviate thirst, always remember to look for causes that may be reversible. Failing that, some practical and useful pointers for dealing with thirst are as follows.

◆ Although tasteless, water is the most effective liquid for relieving or preventing thirst, so always keep a supply of cool water within reach and in a cup or vessel that the person can manage.

◆ Because water is tasteless those with cancer may look for other taste experiences; be alert to this and don't be afraid to try new drinks. Recently, a patient of mine took to lime drinks, having never tried them before.

◆ We are creatures of habit, so if tea and coffee have been the preferred drinks in health they may be sought and appreciated in times of illness. Remember, however, tastes can change.

◆ Alcohol in moderation is fine but it is a mild diuretic so it may be good for the palate but not so good for alleviating thirst.

◆ Cool rather than warm/hot fluids are more soothing for a dry or inflamed throat.

◆ As with food, small amounts of fluid at frequent intervals are generally better than a larger volume all at once. The latter may increase the risk of nausea and vomiting.

◆ Some people like to suck ice. Try ordinary ice or small ice blocks made with Coca-Cola (often recommended by palliative care nurses), other soft drinks, cordials and fruit drinks. This is a tasty and less clinical way of supplementing fluids.

◆ Drinking through a straw or off a spoon may be easier for those too weak to hold or manage a glass or cup.

Intravenous and subcutaneous infusions

As a person becomes weaker and drowsier and less able to drink, fluid intake is reduced and the problems of dry mouth and thirst increase accordingly. At this point, you may wonder about the place of an intravenous infusion to replace fluids and prevent thirst and dehydration.

For those not familiar with the technology, an intravenous infusion involves the insertion of a cannula (thin plastic tube) into a vein and running saline (salt) or dextrose (sugar) solutions through it to replace lost fluids or prevent dehydration. More recently, it has been found that inserting a cannula into the tissues directly beneath the skin and running fluids into this space (subcutaneous infusion) is technically easier and equally effective in replacing fluids. Unlike the intravenous route, antibiotics, vitamins and many drugs cannot be administered via this subcutaneous route.

So what is the place of a subcutaneous or intravenous infusion (from here, referred to simply as a 'drip') in people who are too weak or drowsy to swallow? It would seem that thirst and other symptoms of dehydration can only get worse in this situation and that a drip is the ideal and, in fact, the only thing to do. A little more detail may clarify the situation, dispel the misconceptions and help you formulate your own views.

What symptoms other than thirst occur with dehydration?

Dehydration is a clinical term used when someone is 'dry'. Thirst is the most common and the earliest symptom. Others such as weakness, poor concentration, lethargy and confusion may occur, but only when dehydration is marked. The latter symptoms may also result from severe illness so do not automatically assume dehydration is the cause.

Will a drip ease thirst in someone unable to drink?

No. The only way thirst can be eased is by moistening the mouth and lips with cool liquids. No amount of intravenous or subcutaneous fluids will relieve thirst. If a drip is used, intensive mouth care is still mandatory (see later in chapter).

Will a drip prolong life?

If the illness is so advanced as to interfere with swallowing, death is more likely to result from the illness than lack of fluids. A drip will not prolong life in this situation.

Will a drip make a dying person feel any better?

No. Most if not all the symptoms (thirst excluded) are likely to be a result of the cancer (or other life-threatening illness) and so will not improve with a drip.

Can a drip make matters worse?

It may not make things worse but the increased volume of fluids may introduce several new problems that further complicate care. These problems include frequent urination, which in some instances may create a need for a catheter to prevent incontinence of urine. There is also an increased risk of skin breakdown from fluid accumulating in the tissues beneath the skin (oedema) and an increased risk of chest infections because of fluid accumulating in the lungs. Rattly breathing at the time of death is also more common in those who have a drip.

Given these facts, a drip is rarely if ever used in those who are dying. It does not prolong life or relieve thirst and can introduce new and troublesome symptoms.

How to relieve thirst

As already mentioned, the best and easiest way to alleviate thirst in someone who is unable to drink is to keep the mouth and tongue moist. If the person is awake and strong enough to swallow, small amounts of fluids can be given via a straw or by spoon. Small chips of ice to suck are a useful and soothing way to supplement fluids. The resulting fluid intake is relatively small and falls far short of daily requirements but should be enough to keep the mouth moist and relieve thirst. Remember, the goal is not to achieve full fluid replacement but to give enough liquid to ease thirst.

If a person is unconscious and unable to swallow, the mouth can be kept moist by using artificial saliva sprays or by injecting a small volume of water (1–2 ml) into the mouth via a syringe. This fluid is run in slowly and directly onto the tongue or between the inside of the bottom lip and the lower gum. This volume of fluid administered regularly (every 30–60 minutes during the day and less frequently at night) is large enough to keep the mouth moist and small enough to be absorbed from the mouth without the need to swallow. If necessary, a nurse can also show you how to clean the mouth and keep it moist by using damp swabs. This can be done in combination with any or all of the above measures.

Whether to use a drip in someone dying of cancer may depend on much more than the medical facts. Factors such as cultural, religious and spiritual beliefs, customs and tradition often come into play and must always be respected. Let me illustrate with the examples of Joseph and Tsung.

Joseph had been admitted to the hospice for the relief of pain associated with cancer of the liver. The cancer was far advanced and, although the pain was quickly controlled, Joseph's condition deteriorated rapidly. He was dying and both he and his family were informed of this at a bedside meeting. In the space of one week Joseph became increasingly drowsy and ultimately unconscious. As he was unable to swallow, his mouth care was intensified and pain relief continued. Joseph appeared to be very comfortable.

His wife was distraught and initially I attributed this to grief about her husband's impending death, but as we spoke it became clear there was more to her distress. Both she and Joseph had strong spiritual values that included a belief in reincarnation. They believed that to die in a state of 'dehydration' would seriously compromise the reincarnation process. She wondered if there was something that could be done. Putting my medical prejudice aside, I mentioned an infusion which she readily and happily embraced. Joseph died two days after a subcutaneous infusion had been commenced and his wife, though grieving, was much more at peace about the way he died.

Tsung was an elderly Chinese woman, dying from cancer of the stomach. She had been cared for at home by a large and loving family until she fell and broke her hip. Severe pain necessitated admission to the hospice and an increased dose of morphine. Her condition deteriorated and, while the family could accept the inevitability of her death, they wished to demonstrate their love and respect for all she had done by continuing to offer her sustenance. They asked that we not only start an infusion but that vitamins be added to the infusion to ensure she was not vitamin-deficient. It made no medical sense but it was culturally and personally important to the family that this should be done. Accordingly, an intravenous infusion containing vitamins was commenced and continued to the time of her death several days later.

Bowel care

You may have noticed that in caring for someone who is unwell a lot of emphasis is put on 'the bowels'. Constipation can be a very real and painful problem for anyone, particularly those who are weak and bed-bound. Chronic illness, altered eating habits, reduced food and fluid intake and inactivity combine to make constipation a common complaint among those who are dying.

Surprisingly, a regular bowel motion is just as normal for someone who is unwell and eats very little (or nothing at all) as it is for those who are healthy. The reason is that the bulk of a bowel motion comes from two sources—the residue of what we eat and the natural shedding of cells that line the full extent of the bowel. These cells are shed and renewed on a daily basis and, given the length of the bowel and the number of cells involved, their contribution to the size of a bowel motion is quite substantial.

There is no precise definition for constipation and what one person may label 'constipation' another may not. So constipation is relative but can be said to exist if someone's bowels do not open as often as is normal for them, or if the act of trying to pass a bowel motion is painful, or if after passing a motion a feeling of incomplete emptying remains. The belief that someone's bowels should open every day is therefore erroneous but anything less than three times a week may be a problem.

The chances of constipation are extremely high in the cancer population, not only for the reasons mentioned above but also because of the effects of morphine. Morphine and most pain relievers are constipating so preventive measures are almost always necessary. There is no strong pain reliever that does not cause constipation and so it is always going to be a problem if pain relief is required. Morphine and preparations containing codeine, such as Panadeine Forte, are probably the worst offenders. Morphine has a particularly bad reputation for causing constipation—I liken it to cement, as it can cause the bowel motion to set like concrete if it is 'left too long'. Some of the newer analgesics are not as constipating and, while their pain-relieving qualities may not be as good, they can be used if constipation is obstinate. Your doctor or palliative care nurse can advise you further about these matters.

Morphine or not, any ill person whose lifestyle and eating habits have altered is at risk of constipation and may benefit from preventive measures. Unfortunately, many of the recommendations given to 'healthy' people (e.g. increased intake of fluids and dietary fibre and increased activity) may be difficult if not impossible to implement in those who are unwell. Friends and health care professionals will all have their favourite recipes. I regularly recommend kiwi fruit (one or more per day), prunes and Bekunis tea. If these and other simple measures fail to prevent constipation your loved one may (will, if morphine is on the list of medications) need to resort to laxatives.

The range of laxatives is enormous suggesting (correctly) that one is no better than another. To make matters worse, most of them are fairly mild and the number of tablets or volume of liquid required to do the job (excuse the pun) often reach prohibitive proportions. Laxatives are not free of side effects either and must always be used in the recommended dose. The most frequently prescribed laxatives are Coloxyl tablets, with or without senna, and liquid preparations such as Actilax, Duphalac and Sorbilax. The liquid preparations are sickly sweet and may cause nausea. They also require a good intake of fluid (at least 1000–1500 ml/day) if they are to work and this may not be possible with someone who is ill. Coloxyl with senna is probably the best of a bad lot but senna can, in large doses, cause colic and should be avoided in those with a history of 'bowel blockages'.

A diagnosis of constipation should be easy to make, but it remains one of the most frequently overlooked and misdiagnosed problems in people who are sick and dying. Apart from the obvious discomfort, constipation can cause pain in the lower abdomen, nausea, vomiting, difficulty in passing urine (yes, urine) and very occasionally restlessness and confusion. So keep a record of when the bowels open and tell the doctor or nurse if the bowels have not worked for several days. They will make their own assessment, which generally involves a few questions, a feel of the abdomen and, occasionally, an internal examination through the anus.

You might consider an internal examination intrusive and

unnecessary in a person who is so sick. Intrusive yes, unnecessary no. A diagnosis of constipation can be difficult to make, and an internal examination is often the best way to be sure. Any delay in the diagnosis and treatment of constipation can result in unnecessary and sometimes severe pain. The examination is not painful but is often described as uncomfortable. I imagine it to be more painful to one's dignity. It is not done routinely but only when there is some doubt about the diagnosis or about the best way to treat the constipation. The examination is done with the person in bed and takes only a few seconds.

If the examination confirms constipation, suppositories or enemas are commonly used to rectify the problem. These steps are followed for the not so sick person and also for those who are dying. It might seem unnecessary to resort to such measures in the dying but, whether they are conscious or not, people still feel pain and discomfort from constipation and need the appropriate treatment if they are to settle. In these circumstances pain often manifests as restlessness, particularly in those who are unable to communicate, and will only get worse if not treated. So, if ever your dying relative becomes restless or agitated, do not be surprised if the doctor or nurse raises the possibility of constipation or a full bladder (see below).

Bladder care

Difficulty or an inability to pass urine (the latter is called *urinary retention*) is an infrequent complication of illness but is much more likely to occur in certain forms of cancer, notably cancer of the prostate. Urinary retention can result in severe abdominal pain and will generally require some form of intervention such as a catheter. The problem is frequently overlooked, as it is not unusual for someone with this complication to pass (dribble) very small amounts of urine and this often diverts attention away from the possibility of a blockage. In reality, this is an overflow situation and the key symptoms are worsening abdominal pain, an inability to pass urine or the ability to pass only a few drops at a time. If any of these symptoms occur, always report them to the palliative care team as early as possible. If a catheter is required, it can usually be inserted at home. If there is a high risk of urinary retention, a urinary catheter may be recommended as a precautionary measure. There are obviously benefits and drawbacks to doing this so the decision must be made carefully.

A catheter is inserted via the penis in men and via the urethra in women; in both instances this is referred to as a *urethral catheter*. Local anaesthetic renders the procedure relatively pain-free and the relief that follows quickly atones for any discomfort associated with the catheter's insertion. Much less frequently, the catheter will be inserted through the lower abdomen. This is called a *supra-pubic catheter* and is employed if previous attempts at inserting a urethral catheter have been difficult or when a catheter is required for a long period of time.

When a person is drowsy, unconscious or too weak to use a toilet or bedpan the most common scenario is urinary incontinence. Inability to control the flow of urine can result in embarrassment and wet beds. Here we have a situation where comfort has to be delicately balanced against dignity. The inability to control one's bladder and bowels and the indignity that goes with this is one of the biggest concerns most people have about dying. They may accept or resign themselves to the fact they are dying, but the loss of control over vital functions is another matter. Knowing someone else will have to attend to this is a constant source of worry and embarrassment. I have no simple answers to help you but in the same situation most of us find the following words (or something similar) comforting: 'We love you, and while we know you are embarrassed, we want to care for you (at home) even if that means wiping your bottom and changing a wet bed.' Knowing that family can do it, and choose to do it, goes a long way towards easing a dying person's concern.

There are many aids to help with urinary incontinence. Most of these are available for use at home (as well as in the hospice/hospital) and can be obtained through the community or palliative care nurses. The nurses are the best people to advise you on all aspects of bladder care, so take time to talk to them even if there is no problem. It is better to be prepared.

You might think that urine output would diminish and wet beds be rare in someone who is unable to drink or drinks very little. Prepare yourself for a surprise. People continue to pass reasonable amounts of urine for quite some time after they stop drinking. This is because the body is like a sponge and contains an extraordinary amount of water even in those with a poor fluid intake. Apart from causing embarrassment, wet beds are unpleasant and uncomfortable, irritate the skin and increase the risk of skin breakdown and pressure areas. While prevention may not always be possible, a prompt change of bed linen and pyjamas helps preserve skin integrity as well as dignity.

We are conditioned not to wet the bed so a full bladder is one of many things that can wake a person, sick or healthy, from sleep. If the person is deeply unconscious, they may not wake but may become restless and start to groan. Restlessness in someone previously comfortable or asleep suggests some form of discomfort or pain. A full bladder and a wet bed are two of the many possible causes. So, rather than reaching for a booster dose of morphine or extra sedation, look for a cause and if you do not find one and the restlessness persists call for professional help.

Skin care and pressure areas

As a person's health deteriorates the amount of time spent in bed or a chair increases dramatically and, for someone who has lost weight, these natural and seemingly innocuous positions can present special problems. The fragility of the skin and loss of skin elasticity and tissue padding make weight-bearing areas particularly susceptible to damage. The problem is compounded by weakness that may limit a person's ability to change position and relieve pressure. So when someone is ill and confined to bed or chair, the skin over weight-bearing areas such as buttocks, sacrum, hips, heels and elbows is prone to damage. The result can be a breakdown of normal skin integrity, leading to tears or ulcers, both of which are called pressure areas. These pressure areas may be small or large and are often painful and debilitating. They are prone to infection which results in more pain and significantly delays healing.

The earliest warning sign of a pressure area is redness in one or more of the sites mentioned above. If you notice this or anything worse, tell the community nurse or doctor immediately. The earlier the problem is treated the more likely it is to heal, with less pain and fewer complications. In the earliest stages treatment may involve only repositioning, but dressings and sometimes pain relief are necessary once the skin is broken. The dressings are usually done by the nurses. The frequency of the dressings depends on the site and size of the damaged skin. The nurses will also show you how best to reposition your loved one. These positions are often hard to maintain. They are less comfortable than lying on one's back and often compromise a person's independence. How strictly you enforce the repositioning does therefore depend on circumstances. The overall comfort of the person in the bed should always take precedence.

Prevention is, of course, better than cure and I recommend you speak to the nurses about how this can be done. Depending on the circumstances, pressure areas may be difficult or near impossible to prevent and may appear despite the best care. So do not blame yourself if one or more appear. The following precautionary measures are often recommended:

◆ correct choice of bedding, mattress and chair (the nurse or occupational therapist can advise on this);

◆ correct undercovers for sacrum and heels (e.g. sheepskin rug, boots);

- ◆ regular change of position;
- ◆ keeping susceptible areas clean and dry;
- ◆ rubbing the susceptible areas with appropriate creams as recommended by chemist or nurse;
- ◆ changing wet or moist bed linen and pyjamas as soon as it is noted.

Mouth care

The problems of thirst and dry mouth have been discussed earlier in this chapter under the headings of Fluids and How to relieve thirst.

Oral thrush (also called *monilia*) is one of the most overlooked infections in those who are dying. It may be encountered at any time in the course of a serious illness but is much more common in the later stages. Thrush is a fungal infection, resulting from the same organism that causes thrush in babies. It appears as white plaques anywhere within the mouth but is most commonly seen on the roof of the mouth. It can be easily missed if you only glance in the mouth; careful inspection with a good torch is required if you suspect or wish to exclude the problem. It is more common in those who have been or are still taking antibiotics or cortisone (dexamethasone, prednisolone and prednisone). Thrush causes few early symptoms but left untreated will result in a very sore throat, making swallowing difficult and painful. I have seen many people who were unable to swallow food or fluids simply because of thrush.

Many agents can be used to treat this condition but the most popular are Nilstat or Mycostatin drops. They are more effective than alternatives such as lozenges; to be effective, lozenges need to dissolve and this is virtually impossible in someone with a dry mouth. The drops may sting a little when first used but this is a reflection of the underlying inflammation and is not due to the drops. The drops should be swished around the mouth and kept there as long as possible before being swallowed or spat out. The drops are yellow in colour and will often stain the tongue. This is nothing to worry about. As thrush is often present under dentures it is important to give these a good soak in bicarbonate solution at least once a day. If the thrush is stubborn it may be advisable to leave the dentures out for a good part of the day and at night or, if preferred, for one hour after the drops have been installed.

Some doctors and nurses also use bicarbonate mouthwashes routinely, but this is not really necessary. I reserve it mainly for dentures or if the thrush is not improving with drops alone. Special antifungal tablets are available for the more severe forms of thrush, particularly in those who do not respond to the usual local treatment(s).

Other infections are far less common but I will mention mouth ulcers and gingivitis because they are painful, particularly mouth ulcers. Like thrush they can be difficult to diagnose, so ask your doctor to review the situation if your loved one complains of a painful throat or mouth. Very rarely, a mumps-like infection can occur when the salivary glands in front of the ears swell and become painful. This is not mumps but results in symptoms and signs very similar to that once common childhood infection. It is due to a bacterial infection (mumps is due to a virus) and settles with regular antibiotics and mouth care.

As health deteriorates and fluid intake is reduced, a person may find it increasingly difficult to swallow tablets and it is not unusual to discover them untouched on the bedside table or partly dissolved in the mouth. If this is the case, you can ask the doctor to review the medication, as all except those given for pain and symptom relief can now be ceased. Those that are necessary can usually be given by another route—for example, injection under the skin (subcutaneous)—thereby reducing the tablet burden without compromising pain or symptom control.

The final word on mouth care concerns dentures, which by this time are usually ill fitting and may be more of a problem than an asset. The decision to leave them in or out is obviously up to the individual and appearances as much as comfort will influence the choice. If people are concerned about appearances, they may be happy to leave them out most of the time and put them in only when visitors arrive.

Wound care

Open wounds, skin ulceration and pressure areas should be inspected daily, kept clean and dry and covered with a protective dressing. Exposing simple wounds to direct sunlight for one or more hours a day can be beneficial but is of questionable value if the wound is infected or contains dead or necrotic tissue or tumour. It is best to keep these wounds covered. This is partly for cosmetic reasons but also to shield the wound from flies that might be attracted.

Nurturing

 The way care is given can reach the most hidden places.

Dame Cicely Saunders

The supportive care measures I have described so far all deal with physical comfort. While this is undeniably important, there are other equally important aspects of care. Comfort, including the relief of pain, is just one of the basic needs of someone who is dying. The others are a need for purpose or meaning in one's life and the need to maintain relationships. Together these can be viewed as essential CPR for those who are dying, where CPR stands for Comfort, Purpose and Relationships.

These elements of care are not independent of each other and changes in one can have positive or negative effects on the others. For example, it is not unusual to find that purpose in life and dignity are restored once pain is controlled. Similarly, someone may complain of 'pain' when other aspects of their life or relationships are compromised. This interrelationship between body, mind and spirit is well known and the combination of physical pain, mental anguish and existential searching, so often seen in the dying, is usually referred to as total pain or *suffering*.

Circumstances determine the relative importance of physical, mental and existential pain but in the context of palliative care it seems that physical pain, when present, overrides all other needs. So, one of the goals of palliative care is, whenever possible, first to relieve or ease somatic pain. In so doing, we not only improve comfort and the quality of the person's life but also help restore dignity and purpose, and allow nurturing relationships to resume.

Visits

In the context of ill health, visits form a very important part of social interaction and are often the only avenue a dying person has of maintaining contact with colleagues, friends and even family. Those who are dying frequently lose interest in television, newspapers and local events and, as their world contracts, the only contact between them and the outside is family and friends that visit. Visits are also a way for people to show they care and, ill as their relative/friend may be, the significance of a visit is never lost. People who are dying seek genuine human contact and this genuineness is reflected not only in the frequency of visits, but also in their quality.

Alternatively, it can become a source of concern when a sick person realises ·that friends have stopped visiting or phoning. Circumstances may play a big part in this, but so often visits and phone calls from friends and colleagues just dry up. This is always painful and may add to the feeling of alienation that dying people experience.

Visits can also bring their own problems. Visitors may stay too long, come more often than seems necessary, say inappropriate things or make unrealistic statements. It is not unreasonable for you, as the carer, to ask people to ring days rather than minutes before they come, not only as a matter of courtesy but also to check whether your relative/friend is up to taking visitors. Most visitors will understand if it is not okay or if the visit needs to be cancelled at the last moment. Asking potential visitors to ring also allows you to exert some discretion and select only those you think should visit. It can be difficult for you to say no, but if your loved one is too sick or exhausted or wishes not to see certain people those visits will only add to their distress.

If the timing and circumstances are okay, let visitors know how long they can stay without tiring your relative/friend unduly and ask them to keep to that time. Also, suggest they be alert to what is happening: if the sick person looks tired or is dropping off to sleep, or if other visitors arrive, these may be cues to leave earlier rather than later. Most visitors are unsure how long they should stay—guidelines are often gratefully received and could protect you from the embarrassing situation of asking them to leave.

During visits it is not unusual for friends or relatives to ask if there is some way they can help. As a carer you may, for a multitude of reasons, decline this initial offer. You may feel it is your duty to do everything, you may be embarrassed about accepting help, believe acceptance indicates you are not coping or you may not want 'to put others to the trouble'. Whatever the reason, it is an offer you should not pass up. Not only will it relieve you of some of the more tedious chores, it will free you to spend more quality time with your loved one, family or simply alone. Do not ask too much of yourself or expect that you can take on the difficult task of caring without outside help. We all have our limits and it is better to live within these limits rather than stretch ourselves to breaking point. You, your loved one and your family will all benefit from offers of outside help.

With this in mind, have a list of chores that others can do and, if they do not ask, take courage and ask them. This is not only liberating for you—it can also be deeply rewarding for others to know they can be of help and that you trust them enough to ask. Tasks may include shopping, cooking a meal once a week, doing the washing, vacuuming the house, mowing lawns, gardening, spending time with your loved one while you shop, go for a walk or watch a movie. These requests should not be confined only to this time of caregiving. They are just as helpful and rewarding in the weeks and months following your loved one's death.

Presencing: tips for visitors

Being really present with someone who is dying is not a skill many of us possess. 'Presencing' is a term used to indicate when someone is fully aware of the moment, hears what is being said, does not look for answers or solutions, respects the value of silence and speaks from their heart. It is a tall order but time is precious for those who are dying; to waste time and words on meaningless conversation is thoughtless and can add to a person's suffering. People who are dying dispense with superficial distractions and focus only on what is truly important. Grahame Jones says, 'Let the healthy talk of illness, let the sick speak of more important things.'

The biggest dilemma that people face when visiting someone who is unwell is, what do I say? There is no simple answer nor is there a quick and easy way to learn. To enter with plans about what to say is often counterproductive as this is usually done with our own welfare in mind rather than that of the one we are visiting. So, threatening as it may seem, enter with an open mind and an open heart and allow the conversation to flow rather than be steered and controlled by you. The following points may help.

◆ Listening is more important than speaking.
◆ Be aware of how you feel and try not to let this become your agenda (the story of Helen that follows will illustrate what I mean by this).

◆ Your body language will mean much more to the ill person than any of the words you use. So sit rather than stand, near rather than far away, make good eye contact and be fully aware of what is happening with the person you are visiting.

◆ Be real and authentic. Your job is not to try to make the person feel better nor to make conversation. They know if you are playing this game and will go along with it, at their own expense. If you do this it is often because you are uncomfortable and unsure about what to say. Being real and authentic is to say 'I don't know what to say' when that is how you feel.

◆ Don't be afraid of silences. They are a time of processing, a time when the mind goes quiet and buried thoughts and emotions rise to the surface.

◆ If you say something you wished you had not said, say so. Such honesty is liberating and much better than a quick change of subject.

◆ Avoid false claims such as 'You look so much better' (when they don't). They know when you are being 'nice'.

◆ People don't change because they are dying and nor should you so, bearing in mind all that has been said, relate to the person as you always have in the past.

The American author and caregiver Ram Dass recounts the following story from one of the workshops of Dr Elisabeth Kübler Ross.

Helen was a young woman in her mid-thirties. She was a widow with two children, aged 7 and 9 years. Cancer of the breast had been diagnosed two years earlier and, despite multiple operations, chemotherapy and radiotherapy, the disease had spread to her liver, lungs and bones and she was expected to die in a matter of months. Although very thin and weak she had decided to attend one of Elisabeth Kübler-Ross's workshops.

During this workshop she asked those present how they

would feel if they came to visit her. Most said they would feel sadness. Sad that a mother of two children was dying so young, or that she would not see her kids grow up, or sad for the children. Others said they would feel anxious about what to say and others would feel angry that someone in her situation should be so afflicted. After a while, Helen said that if any of these people came to visit they would be so weighed down by their own grief there would be little room for her pain. The visit may help them but it would have been of little benefit to her.

The moral of this story, which is particularly pertinent to carers and the immediate family, is that it is very hard to be there for someone if you are weighed down by your own grief. 'When we are too full of our own suffering we cannot accept the suffering of others', says Merrill Collett in his book *At Home with Dying*. Not only is it hard to be there, but this form of suffering can lead you to distance yourself physically and/or emotionally from your loved one at a time when you both need each other. If this situation continues for any length of time, the resulting distress further compounds each other's grief and the ramifications may spill over to involve other family members as they take sides with one or other of the aggrieved. Depending on the degree of suffering and how entrenched the behaviour is, the situation may be resolved by open and honest communication or may require the expertise of a counsellor.

 I cannot know myself except through the intermediary of another person.

J.-P. SARTRE

Precious normality

One of the very sad things about dying is that the closer someone is to death the more likely they are to be treated as a patient rather than a person. In the context of illness, treatments, tests, visits to doctors and visits by nurses all add up and rob sick and dying people of normal living. Grahame Jones described what it is like when he said, 'What I detest is how effectively the procedure of the treatment robs me of my precious normality and seriously affects my morale.'

Illness does rob people (patient and relatives) of precious normality and, while you may have little control over this, it is important that you and your loved one do not become victims in the process. Retain as much as you can of what is normal in your life irrespective of what else is happening around you. Not only should you seek to retain what is normal, you should guard it as you would anything of value. There are many obstacles in the way but the value of such an investment makes it worthwhile for you, the carer, your family and for the one who is dying.

What is normal for the person dying is something that you as relative, carer or friend would know and can therefore maintain and guard. For some it may be reading and, when that is no longer possible, they may like to be read to. For others it may be listening to music, watching videos, doing crosswords, sitting in a much loved garden, emailing friends, writing poetry, having a few drinks or going to the 'local' once a week.

Most important of all is the maintenance (as much as the illness allows) of the previous patterns of intimacy, sensual and sexual sharing. Illness may weaken the body but the desire for closeness and intimacy is never lost. Do not let illness or the fear of causing pain (physical or emotional) come between you and the one you love. If the one who is dying is your spouse or partner, whatever the time of day or night, do not be afraid to hop into bed with them, cuddle them, caress them and be as sensual as circumstances allow. Protect such intimate moments by taking the phone off the hook and putting a 'do not disturb' sign on the front door. Everything else can wait. For all others, closeness is something that must be respected but not abused. Maintain a level of closeness similar to that which existed before the illness. Anything more or less is not only artificial but also patronising.

For the one who is sick, what is normal may no longer be possible. Going back to full-time work or doing chores around the house may be normal but totally unrealistic. Common sense must prevail and often the realisation that they can no longer do these things is painful and confronting. Rather than excluding normality, such a realisation introduces a measure of reality and directs the person to invest more time in things that are normal but possible.

Creating a nurturing physical environment is a useful and meaningful exercise for you to engage in with your loved one as it not only gets priorities in order but can be a healing and cathartic process for both. Some peripheral but related things to consider are these:

◆ Protect and maintain a normal home environment by censoring any unnecessary or unwanted visits to and from other people.

◆ Prepare for dying but not at the expense of living.

◆ Have the dying person spend most of their day in the place they prefer, doing what they prefer.

◆ Get full value out of their favourite clothing, CDs or books.

◆ Within reason maintain your usual routines and habits.

◆ Keep a regular check on needs and preferences.

◆ Keep the medical paraphernalia in another room if at all possible.

◆ Make adjustments to 'precious normality' depending on the need and state of your loved one.

Jessie was resident in a nursing home for six months prior to her death. For all but the last two weeks of her life she was active and alert and wanted her room to be a reflection of the family home she had lived in for 40 years. She had a clock on the wall, photos of her family and grandchildren, a TV to watch her favourite programs on, a radio to listen to at the dead of night and frequent visits from all the family. It became her home away from home.

Following the first of two strokes, Jessie was unable to speak but she was clearly afraid and wanted her family to be with her as much as time allowed. A greeting and parting kiss were no longer sufficient. She needed hugs, cuddles and kisses and no amount of contact was too much. A second stroke one week later rendered her unconscious. She did not respond to the spoken word but seemed to rouse whenever she was held. The TV and the hoards of visitors now seemed out of place and the family felt she would at this time in her life want only her immediate family around. A roster was drawn up and from that moment on Jessie was never alone. She died just as she would have wished, surrounded by her mementos and with her family by her side.

Caring for the carer

Time may be in short supply for the one who is dying and so their wish to make every moment and every contact quality time is not unreasonable. This is easier said than done, particularly for the carer. To be on call, fully aware and present throughout a person's illness can be extraordinarily hard, not only because of the physical task but because of the emotional effort required. Such commitment is often beyond one person's capacity. Be realistic in what you can do and don't be afraid to ask for help. Acknowledge what is going on inside you and, if necessary, find somebody you can confide in. Feelings of frustration, helplessness and anger are not uncommon and are very normal in this situation. You are the primary carer and unless you care for yourself it is very hard to care for someone else, even when that person is one you love dearly.

Survival for you as a carer involves preserving some of your own precious normality, whether that is an afternoon nap, a weekly game of golf or bowls, a morning with friends, unencumbered shopping or going to the movies. These things should not be regarded as luxuries that you can no longer afford but essentials in preserving your own emotional and physical well-being. They are as essential as regular meals and sleep. Looking after people who are dying can be compared to running a marathon. The prime goal of any runner is to finish and that is more likely if they pace themselves from the start. As conditions change, the way they run the race will also change. And that is how it should be for you as the carer. Go slowly at the start, adjust your pace depending on the circumstances and aim to be there in one piece at the end of your race.

In the men's marathon at the 1968 Mexico City Olympics the last runner to finish entered the stadium one hour after the winner had crossed the line. He was bruised and battered from an earlier fall and hobbled exhausted across the finishing line. His finish was greeted with loud applause and when asked why he persisted when so many others had dropped out, he said 'My country did not send me to start the race but to finish.' This wisdom can be applied to many things in life but no more so than the situation you now find yourself in.

6   States of consciousness

To die, to sleep;
To sleep! Perchance to dream: ay, there's the rub;
For in that sleep of death what dreams may come,
When we have shuffled off this mortal coil.

WILLIAM SHAKESPEARE, *Hamlet, Act III, Scene I*

*a*s a palliative care doctor I have been closely associated with the care of many people who have died. The experience of caring for your loved one may lead you to wonder how anyone could do this type of work. Rest assured, you are not the only one who thinks this way. Whenever the topic of work comes up in conversation, as it often does, there is always a distinct silence when I tell people I work in palliative care. If not their words, it is their body language that gives them away. They are clearly taken aback. If the opportunity arises for me to ask what it is about palliative care that makes them feel uncomfortable, most touch on the elements of sadness and fear. There is no denying those emotions go with the territory. But what they and others like them fail to appreciate is that in caring for the dying we get to know them and their family intimately and that the work takes us into the 'deep shadows of mystery and the unknown' (Thomas Moore, *Care of the Soul*).

This mystery is death. Until relatively recent times, death had great religious significance and was considered a mystical event, even though it carried with it all the same emotions we feel today. A scientific and secular revolution over the past 100 years has seen this mystical element seriously challenged, with death now reduced to the biological equivalent of an 'amen' at the end of a litany of physiological changes and medical interventions. It is ironic to realise that, as death takes on more of a biological status, extraordinary and unusual things are being increasingly reported at and around this time. These events, such as the near death experience (NDE), defy rational explanation and do, in their own way, challenge the contemporary reductionist view we have formed of death.

This chapter looks at some of these strange and extraordinary events. While they do not say anything definitive about death or what follows they may serve to reinforce the sense of mystery and the unknown that Thomas Moore spoke of.

Unconsciousness

Part of the mystery is the so-called unconscious state. Unconsciousness is a state that the majority of people with cancer or, indeed, anyone with a chronic illness will go through before they die. We recognise it and label a person 'unconsciousness' when they no longer respond to the spoken word and make no purposeful movement. No one really understands what happens or indeed if anything happens in the mind of someone who is unconscious but the name suggests that nothing of importance takes place.

When we talk about states of consciousness most people are familiar with the two extremes—consciousness and unconsciousness—and naturally believe one is the exact opposite of the other. If we accept consciousness to be a state of awareness in which we assimilate information, process it and respond appropriately, then unconsciousness, by definition, should be a state where there is no awareness, no processing of information and an inability to take appropriate action.

Arnold Mindell in his book on *Coma* says, 'There are powerful and dramatic events trying to unfold themselves in comatose states and nothing happens in coma that is not trying to happen to people all the time.' Such a comment flies in the face of our conventional understanding of coma (unconsciousness) and, if true, would greatly alter our thoughts about death and the way we relate to and care for those who are dying.

Many of my patients prefer to die at home and Pam was no exception. She had a long history of bowel cancer that had continued to grow despite various forms of chemotherapy. Her appetite waned, she lost a considerable amount of weight and ultimately weakness confined her to bed. There was little pain and only small doses of morphine were required to keep her comfortable. Slowly, the weakness overcame her mind as well as her body and she changed from being someone who loved to read and interact with family and friends to someone who slept most of the time, and then to not waking at all. Pam had become unconscious.

Pam was so 'deeply unconscious' she did not react when the nurses inserted a catheter into her bladder. After several days of not responding, eating or drinking I unwisely pronounced that death was at hand. I visited the next day and there was no change. The following day I rang to see if Pam was still alive and to my surprise I was told she was not only alive but very much awake. She was eating, drinking champagne and entertaining the family. It was her birthday! There was a dramatic deterioration over the next 24 hours but she was still aware and extremely peaceful. Twenty-four hours later she was once again unconscious and died shortly after.

Stories such as this are not uncommon and certainly challenge the medical profession's long-held belief that unconsciousness, or coma, is a relatively inert interlude on the path between life and death. The mystery deepened when I realised that many of the patients that woke (albeit temporarily) had some awareness of events during their period of unconsciousness. Sometimes, this awareness was minimal but others could remember detail that family and others had forgotten. In Pam's case it is not unreasonable to suggest her period of wakefulness may have been related to her birthday, and that she had some awareness of this even though she had been deeply unconscious for several days before.

Angela's story adds to the mystery and, like many of the experiences encountered around death (or near death), what happened defies rational explanation.

> Angela was 42 when she died of longstanding cancer. She was the mother of two young children so her death was associated with enormous sadness and grief. As is my practice I visited Angela's family later in the day. Her husband Bill was unsettled and asked me to stay awhile. He then told me of something that had shocked and shaken him. Angela's elder sister had become terribly upset because of a long-forgotten memory that came flooding back only hours after her sister's death. She told Bill how Angela, as a young girl, was very ill from septicaemia and that everyone, including the doctors, had expected her to die. Miraculously, she recovered but some time after the event Angela told her sister that, as she lay there unconscious, she heard a voice say she would survive the septicaemia but would die at the age of forty two.

Many similar stories suggest that those who are unconscious are not oblivious to what is happening around them and that the level of awareness may be much greater than we have until now considered possible. Among other things, it indicates how little we know about death and dying and how much we take for granted. This is particularly true for the medical profession, a profession that devotes so much of its time, effort and money to investigating cures but so little to the understanding and treatment of those who are dying. As we will all some day die, this does not make sense. The American physician Eric Krakauer recognised this paradox when he said, 'We as physicians attend to the dying every day but we have not attended to dying itself.'

Awareness during unconsciousness

Awareness during unconsciousness is not just confined to those who are dying. A large study involving 2517 anaesthetised patients, published in 1996 by Drs Philip Merikle and Meredyth Daneman, concluded that information unconsciously perceived during anaesthesia is remembered for many hours and may remain for weeks if the information is personally relevant and meaningful. This form of remembering is unlike the memory that operates in our daily life which we call upon, successfully or unsuccessfully, to help us plan and make decisions. Information perceived during unconsciousness is not so readily available and cannot generally be recalled but can, without our knowing, influence our thoughts and actions. It can be likened to a dream that may influence the way we feel the following day even though there is no memory of it. 'Getting out on the wrong side of the bed' is a good example of this phenomenon!

The mystery and fascination with this subject led me to embark on a study to see whether awareness in people who were unconscious and dying could be documented scientifically. This seemed important, not just from an academic standpoint, but because the findings could have a significant influence on our understanding of the dying process and the way care is delivered during this time. To do this, we used an instrument that recorded brainwave activity and converted the record to a numerical score that accurately reflected the level of awareness. A score of 100 indicates a fully aware or wide-awake state while 0 indicates brain death and therefore no awareness. To set the scene, a level of 50–55 is the score anaesthetists aim for during anaesthesia as the likelihood of recall is extremely low at that level of awareness. A score as low as 40 or as high as 80 may occur during the stages of normal sleep.

After the necessary ethical, patient and family approval we used this instrument to study the level of awareness in twelve people who were dying (ten with cancer, one with cardiac failure and one with AIDS). The study began the moment each person became unconsciousness and continued until the time of death. The results were surprising, to say the least.

The average score at the time of unconsciousness was 55 and just prior to death it was 44. Both these levels are equivalent to a deeply anaesthetised state and suggest little, if any, possibility of awareness. The score, however, did not remain static but undulated, shooting up to 60–80 when people were moved or when they were in pain. In either situation, the increase in awareness was often accompanied by groans and/or frowning. This proves quite categorically that unconscious patients feel pain and their level of awareness increases to almost wakefulness when pain is present. These findings were not altogether surprising—we know pain and discomfort can wake us from the deepest sleep, so it is not unreasonable to expect the same in those who are unconscious. This finding provides a strong argument for continuing pain relief in those who are unconsciousness. While this came as no surprise, the observation that similar fluctuations in awareness also occurred in the absence of pain was unexpected.

Alberto was the first person we monitored in this study. At the time the machine was connected he was deeply unconscious and unresponsive even when turned. His reading was 40. No sooner had I connected the machine, the bedside phone rang and the level immediately jumped to 65, suggesting that the ring had at least registered in his mind. Seeing this, his mother asked whether the same response might occur if she spoke to her son. Not sure of what to expect and fearing disappointment if there was no response, I hesitatingly agreed and she bent over and whispered into his ear. Again the reading shot up to 65 and, while no physical changes were noted, the reading remained at that level for the brief time she spoke to him and a little while after.

This increased awareness in response to sound was a reasonably common but not universal finding. It supports the widely held belief that hearing is the last sense to go in those dying and that this sense is preserved late into the unconscious period. Even more startling was the occasion when one of the subjects woke from a deeply unconscious state, communicated with her family for approximately 30 minutes and then lapsed back into unconsciousness. Her level prior to waking was 55, fluctuated between 80 and 100 while she was lucid and then fell back to 55. I spoke to the family shortly after and they said their mother woke and said goodbye to them all. Interestingly, all the family were present at this time. She died several days later.

There were two other important observations from this study.

◆ There were regular and cyclical fluctuations in the levels, unassociated with pain, and with no obvious change in the person's state of awareness. The patterns were remarkably similar to what is found during normal dreaming and leads me now to believe that dreams occur even when people are deeply unconscious.

◆ At the time of death the reading dropped dramatically from an average of 44 to zero. This was not unexpected. What was surprising was a brief awakening, lasting 10–20 seconds, that preceded death in many of the subjects. During this period the reading rose to 90 or thereabouts before falling dramatically to zero.

So what does all this mean? Put simply, it confirms that unconsciousness is not an inert state and is definitely not the polar opposite of waking consciousness. If anything, it is probably more akin to sleep. The results also suggest that unconscious patients do assimilate and process information in ways we do not yet fully understand. They dream, feel pain, hear sounds and appreciate voices. This I know. I don't know if anything else is happening or what all this means in the context of death.

The possibility that dreaming can take place in people who are unconscious is of more than academic interest. Michael Kearney, a well known and respected palliative care doctor, has researched the subject of dreams and healing extensively. He believes that dreams help the sick or dying person prepare for death. This being the case, unconsciousness may in fact be a very important step along this path and, like Shakespeare, we can only wonder 'what dreams may come when we have shuffled off this mortal coil'.

Although we know very little about dreaming, evidence now suggests it is a state of consciousness in its own right and not some interesting interlude between sleeping and waking. It is a dynamic state full of activity and potential. Dr Michel Jouvet, one of the foremost researchers on the subject of dreams, made a startling revelation in his latest book, *The Paradox of Sleep—The Story of Dreaming*. His research has shown that the brain is more active and consumes more energy during the phases of REM sleep (dreaming) than during ordinary waking consciousness—that is, when subjects are fully alert. As evidence now suggests that unconscious dying patients also dream, we can assume their brain is just as active during their dreaming phases. Given that other parts of the body are shutting down, this is quite a paradox and raises questions about what is happening in the brain of those who are dying.

The temporary and dramatic increase in awareness at the moment of death is startling but, given what I have just said, it may not be so unusual after all. The experience of those who care for the dying suggests that this awakening prior to death is not an infrequent occurrence. I have witnessed it on many occasions and noticed that these people were staring into space as if looking at something or someone. Whether this is a deathbed vision, part of a dream or a startle response is something we shall discuss shortly.

These findings have major implications for the care we give to those who are dying. It suggests we should relate to them as though they can hear and, whenever it seems appropriate, we should include them in our conversations. I always suggest that people introduce themselves when they enter the room of someone who is unconscious, make some form of physical contact (kiss, touch) and tell the person what they are about to do (e.g. sit for a while). A minimum of words is required, as the dying person may not be capable of assimilating everything, just as you can't when you are in a 'dreamy' state. As with sleep, time does not seem to exist for those who are unconscious so don't be concerned about long gaps in conversation or the hours you are away from the bedside. What seems an age for you is but a fleeting moment for the one who is unconscious.

One reassuring point that came out of the study is that morphine and other medications used appropriately do not, in any significant way, affect awareness levels or any of the normal processes such as dreaming. Levels of awareness have been recorded in two dying people who were on no medication whatsoever. Their results were remarkably similar to those who did receive treatment.

Other states of consciousness

Waking consciousness and unconsciousness are just two of many states of consciousness. Some of the others are:

- sleeping consciousness;
- dreaming consciousness;
- transitional states of consciousness, as with going to sleep or waking;
- consciousness associated with meditation and deep relaxation;
- altered states of consciousness, of which mystical experience, the near death experience (NDE), the out of body experience (OBE) and the deathbed vision (DBV) are good examples.

Near death experiences and deathbed visions

Altered states of consciousness are not infrequent in the context of dying and most commonly occur within hours to weeks of death. During any of these states individuals are fully aware of their own environment, but have an appreciation of things that others cannot see, hear or experience. Sceptics like to call this an hallucination. I believe this is too simple and convenient a label and hope to convince you otherwise.

> Stella had been near to unconscious for several days. I happened to be in the room when she suddenly sat bolt upright and, with eyes fixed on the wall ahead, beamed with delight. I asked her to describe what she was looking at but there was no reply, although she continued to look ahead as though mesmerised. Her daughter arrived about this time but she, like me, could not distract her from what she was experiencing. Despite her glow she looked most unwell and after several minutes she lay back on the bed and died.

These unusual but well publicised experiences occur in the face of death or, in the case of NDEs, with the threat or fear of death (note that NDEs and DBVs are very similar and differ mainly in the matter of survival). Visions, usually of predeceased relatives and/or religious figures, are the most common and pronounced feature of a DBV and this is nearly always accompanied by a sense of joy and peace that is so overwhelming the person often finds it hard to describe. Given the gravity of the situation these emotions seem out of place. A striking feature of the visions is their vividness, so much so that the person may awake from sleep or unconsciousness and be totally absorbed and overwhelmed by what they see. According to Drs Karlis Osis and Erlendur Haaraldsson, authors of one large study, the vision is 'so real that only very very rarely will the person doubt the reality of the apparition'.

When I was eight years of age, I almost drowned. I have few memories of that era but the drowning incident remains very clear. Holding on to a large beach ball, I paddled out into the smooth but deep waters of a lake. As the ball slipped from my grasp and I slid under the water I thought how foolish I had been. When I surfaced, I thrashed around in an unsuccessful attempt to stay afloat. My memory of that struggle is surprisingly vague—surprising, because everything else was and still is so clear. A young couple was walking along the water's edge but they seemed engrossed in conversation and did not see me or hear my sister's call for help. For some reason, I remember thinking they were probably newlyweds and that I should not disturb them during what I felt was an intimate moment. It seems bizarre, but at the time I was more concerned for them than for my own welfare. At that very moment, I was not afraid and felt a peace and serenity the likes of which I have not known since. I seemed acutely aware of all that was outside of me but felt none of the terror that should have accompanied the event.

For the record, I was rescued by one of my brothers who heard my sister's call. I have no memory of being pulled from the water and my next recollection is some time later when I woke to find my parents peering down at me. I have always wondered if this was an NDE, but that is somewhat academic. What is important, at least for me, is the knowledge and first-hand experience of how peaceful dying, or at least drowning, can be.

DBVs and NDEs are not new but the number of reports of NDEs has increased dramatically over the last 40 or 50 years. This surge is probably a result of improvements in resuscitation techniques which have seen many more people survive a life-threatening situation to tell of their experience. Approximately 15–50 per cent of people who come close to death recall having an NDE and 25 per cent of those that die will tell of a DBV beforehand. This latter figure may be artificially low bearing in mind that those who die have fewer opportunities to talk of their experience.

One of the earliest recorded reports of a DBV concerned a young mother who was dying within days of the birth of her first child. Expecting her patient to be distraught, the doctor was stunned by this woman's apparent peace and sought an explanation. The woman's response to her doctor's leading question was 'If you could see what I can see you would understand'.

In an attempt to find out more about DBVs, we contacted the next of kin of patients who had died in our hospice over a three-month period. We were surprised to learn that 23 per cent had either witnessed or been told about a DBV by their now deceased loved one. In all cases, these visions were described by the dying person or seen by the next of kin to be comforting. Comments such as these were common:

- ◆ 'Mum said she had seen many of her deceased relatives.'
- ◆ 'Mum saw different relatives in the room.'
- ◆ 'He saw a person in a white dress holding out her hand.'
- ◆ 'She gazed into the air in front of her, whereupon she seemed happy and content.'

Trent was a young man with recently diagnosed but rapidly advancing cancer. The cancer had spread throughout his bones and caused him considerable pain. Despite frequent courses of radiotherapy and large doses of morphine the pain increased, so much so that admission to hospital became necessary. Adjustments to treatment resulted in some, though not complete, pain relief. Despite large doses of morphine he was lucid at all times. He was a popular and well known personality and his room was always filled with visitors. One evening, his father joined the hordes of people in the room and, as he went to sit on the only empty chair, his son called out, 'Be careful you don't sit on my friend, Dad.' 'What friend?' asked his father, looking at the empty chair. 'My friend, a good friend, who will shortly be taking me away.' Everyone was stunned.

Trent then told those present in the room about this friend who had been there with him for several days.

I never got the opportunity to ask Trent about his invisible friend but, in conversation with his family, it seemed as if this 'friend' was not someone he knew or recognised. He was nonetheless a source of comfort during Trent's final days of life. It would be easy to attribute this to an hallucination or trick of the mind, induced by a perilous state of health or a large dose of morphine. Given his otherwise clear mind and appropriate conversation, this proposition seems unlikely. What is important and what really matters is that, in Trent's eyes, this friend was real and brought a quiet and comforting presence during those difficult last days.

Whatever way it comes, comfort is a blessing, particularly during the last days of life. It is a theme that characterises many a DBV, as the following example illustrates.

Nina was an elderly Italian woman. She had advanced cancer of the uterus and had been admitted to the local hospice from home. She spoke very little English and, because of this and her weakened state, she made no demands on the staff. She appeared withdrawn and sad. The family had asked she not be told she was dying even though her body language suggested she already knew. One day, just after the family arrived for their regular daily visit, they rushed out of her room, grabbed me as I passed by and urged me to give their mother an injection to settle. They said she was agitated and was asking to leave the hospice. She was sitting bolt upright in bed, speaking in her native tongue. Her eyes were fixed on the wall as if she was looking at something but what struck me was the big smile on her face. I asked the family to interpret what Nina was saying. 'I am going on a big holiday, the boat is here, my bags are packed and none of you can come with me.' Although Nina was filled with joy, the family was distraught, as they had interpreted her rambling to mean she wanted to leave the hospice. I explained that she was not asking to leave but was telling her family that the time for her to die had arrived. I encouraged them to sit and allow her to talk about this journey. She died two days later. Following the funeral, the family returned to the hospice to thank us for caring for their mother and for helping them to understand the significance of Nina's vision.

The next case is more bizarre than most, but the message of comfort that eventually comes as Rhonda hears the words 'It's okay' is equally clear. I was very uncertain about what was happening at the time but trusted my intuition and followed the lead set by Rhonda. Like the other examples, it illustrates the sense of mystery that often prevails around the time of death and how easily significant events can be overlooked, reduced to a mere aberration or placated with medication.

Rhonda had been in the hospice for more than a month with cancer of the bowel. The symptoms of pain and vomiting had been difficult to control and persisted despite numerous changes in medication. I saw her late one morning and asked how things were going. She said she was more comfortable and had not vomited for at least 24 hours. She thanked me for my visit and said she planned to have a sleep.

One hour later I was contacted by the nurse to say that Rhonda was very distressed, rigid with pain and requesting an injection to ease the discomfort. Because this was such a contrast to what I had seen earlier I went to see Rhonda before making a decision on treatment. I found her writhing in pain and clutching a heat pack to her stomach. I knelt by her side and asked her to tell me what was happening. To my surprise, she started speaking in a strange way; her words ran into each other and it was difficult to understand everything she said, but the exchange went something like this.

Rhonda: Oh, it is terrible, all the oranges and browns, like waves, oh, oh.

[She was rigid at this time, appeared frightened and clutched the hot pack tightly to her stomach.]

Michael: Is there any place you can go to get away from them?

Rhonda: Yes, yes, the dark blue. It's beautiful.

Michael: Go to it, Rhonda, and wrap yourself in that dark blue.

[Rhonda relaxed but after a short time spoke again: It's back again, all the oranges and browns. She mentioned other colours that I could not quite catch and again she became very agitated.]

Michael: Go back to the dark blue, Rhonda. It is right by you; wrap yourself tightly in the dark blue.

[Again she relaxed.]

Rhonda: Must get that piping; what's it doing here?

Michael: Tell me about the piping.

Rhonda: What is it doing here?

Michael: Is anyone there with you?

Rhonda: Yes, my aunt [whom she named]. She looks thin and old.

Michael: I think she has come to see how you are. Is anyone else there?

Rhonda: Yes, can't be sure but I think it is her mother.

Michael: Ask them what they want.

[Long silence]

Michael: What did they say, Rhonda?

Rhonda: It's okay.

Michael: Yes, it is okay. All you need to do is stay with the blue and they will look after you.

Rhonda: Jam, I need some blackcurrant jam and blackberry jam.

Michael: I don't have any but will water do?

Rhonda: Yes thanks.

[She had a sip, settled and relaxed into sleep.]

During this exchange Rhonda's eyes were mostly closed. I left the room after she had gone to sleep and a volunteer sat with her. She was still asleep when I called back, one and then two hours later. By the third hour the family had arrived and Rhonda had gone to the bathroom for a wash. At the end of the day the nurses reported that Rhonda was pain-free and comfortable. She was lucid and had a good few hours with her family. As I was about to leave, they asked what magic words I had used!

Rhonda died 12 days later having had no further strange episodes. Her death was peaceful, considering the problems associated with her cancer.

These are just a few examples among many that indicate some of the bizarre happenings around death and the comfort dying people can derive from them. It also confirms how little we know or understand about the processes that take place when someone is dying. Much of the current debate surrounds the possible cause of NDEs, DBVs and other altered states of consciousness; while this is important we must not lose sight of the fact that, whatever the cause, the experience and what it means for that person is what really matters. Looking for causes without appreciating the significance of the experience is similar to studying how a flower blossoms without appreciating its essential beauty.

For the person who is dying, the experience has a deep and powerful meaning that can easily be invalidated because it seems obtuse or bizarre to the outsider. Similarly, experiences may be overlooked because they are so subtle. Some of what we label confusion in the dying may in fact be profound experiences that can so easily be lost because we do not tune into the right 'wavelength'. Ram Dass, a well known and respected American psychologist who does a lot of voluntary work for hospices, tells a wonderful story that illustrates this point.

One evening he was contacted by a hospice to see if he could help settle a man who was dying. Despite all manner of medical treatment this man had been 'raving' for days. Ram Dass sat by the man who continued to make unintelligible noises. Ram did not know what was happening or what he should do but after a while decided to imitate the sounds. The noise emanating from the room became much louder and the staff wondered if they had done the right thing in calling for outside help. Ram Dass persisted in imitating the noise and after some time the man turned to him and said, 'So you can see them too?' More of the harmonising followed and the man eventually settled and remained settled until his death.

No one really understands what happens during these altered states of consciousness just as we do not know their cause(s). I have tried to demonstrate that the capacity for awareness in these states is so much greater than most of us would believe possible. It is something of a paradox to realise that a person's consciousness can expand to incorporate these experiences as they and their body die. Some experts suggest that these altered states of consciousness should be called states of superconsciousness, 'super' because of the ability to tune into things that ordinary waking consciousness cannot perceive and therefore rejects.

Our brain is a wonderful organ but it contains and limits consciousness to such a degree that conscious awareness is confined to worldly things. It finds it difficult to include the mystical and the mysterious, including the concept of immortality. In its 'mind's eye' death is final and tells us our consciousness dies with our physical body. The Dutch philosopher Spinoza believed otherwise and 430 years ago, said that true happiness and contentment is contained in *sub specie aeternitatis*—that is, seeing everything from the perspective of eternity.

The more we become attuned to our essential being the more we appreciate the possibility of a disembodied existence and life beyond death. Many people who have had an NDE talk of being able to view their body from afar as if it did not belong to them. They have a real sense of living outside the body and, for many, this state was so appealing they had to make a 'conscious' decision to return. Those who have had an NDE say the experience is indescribable and that it feels more real than life itself. So profound is this effect that most lose all fear of death and see life in a totally different light.

No one can yet say whether these experiences are mere machinations of a dying brain or some transcendental event but, whatever the cause, no one seriously doubts their occurrence. The experiences I have described are hard for us to comprehend and, in not being able to comprehend, there is the danger we might reject them. What we have learnt about unconsciousness is that we know very little about it. Consciousness appears to be always present but the quality of consciousness is not fixed. It is influenced by many factors— some external, such as drugs, anaesthetic agents, illness or accident, and some internal, such as meditation, sleeping or dreaming.

Death and dying also have a profound effect on consciousness and the association with NDEs and DBVs suggests that dying 'fine-tunes' consciousness into frequencies not appreciated by the living. This is very relevant to the care of someone who is dying as they, more than anyone, have the potential to experience what William James called the 'wide field' or expanded states of consciousness. This so-called wide field not only includes NDEs and DBVs but the enigmatic state of unconsciousness. In relation to death, Elisabeth Kübler-Ross says, 'They are not going into nothingness, they're entering another state of being.'

These expanded states of consciousness are not new nor are they confined to the dying. They have been described by many and varied mystical traditions and for centuries have formed part of their spiritual practices. They may also be induced by ritualistic native practices that frequently involve the use of mind-altering substances such as mushrooms. These historical roots have led to a natural conclusion that altered states of consciousness can only be induced, and are not part of a natural state. Recent work and observation have suggested quite the opposite. Stilling the mind with meditation, prayer, prolonged silence or isolation is now known to be just as potent as ritualistic and spiritual practices in inducing altered states of consciousness.

This raises the possibility that a conscious mind that is both active and interactive limits consciousness to a state of cognition, and only when it is switched off by any of the means mentioned above (including sleep) does it allow the 'wider field' of consciousness to permeate. This seems very relevant to dying, particularly when dying includes a period of unconsciousness. Dying introduces physical and mental stillness, social and sensory isolation, conditions known to be conducive to the development of altered states of consciousness. So rather than being unusual, altered states of consciousness, including NDEs and DBVs, should be expected and are, indeed, relatively common among those who are dying. Whether these states are mystical or physiological remains to be determined but their occurrence and significance is now beyond question.

Irrespective of your belief system, I hope what has been said will influence you as much as it has me to be open to the metaphysical and unknown dimensions of death, and to appreciate that more rather than less is happening as death approaches. I hope it also gives you the strength and courage to remain close to the one who is dying, to tune into whatever is happening and to speak to them. A prolonged period of unconsciousness may not be as meaningless as many of us have previously thought. There may be some deeper meaning and hidden reason behind what might appear to be a slow protracted death. If nothing else, the way we care for the dying person who is unconscious bears re-examining.

The best is perhaps what we understand least.

NW CLERK, *A Grief Observed*

7 What happens around the time of death?

The dark and silent river
Pursues through tangled woods a way

HW Longfellow

*t*he tragedy on September 11, 2001 when two fully laden jets crashed into the New York Twin Towers left everyone shocked and dismayed. We grieved individually and collectively but our grief was minuscule compared with the grief felt by those who lost friends and relatives, or by those who were present at 'ground zero'. When we face our own death, lose someone we love or are ourselves at ground zero, only then will we know death and experience its full might, its secrets and its mystery.

In an era where few children die and most adults survive beyond the age of seventy years our idea of death is often nothing more than a cut and paste job, incorporating the many different impressions we acquire from newspapers, radio, TV and film. The concept so formed is far removed from the truth and rarely prepares us for the real thing when it comes along. In his autobiography, *In the Face of Death*, Peter Noll speaks of his own experience of dying and says, 'What we figure out in our heads looks quite different once realised in reality.'

The task of being a carer is demanding and unremitting and the roles you have to fill are many and varied. Over the course of a life-threatening illness the tasks and roles change but the goal of maintaining the best quality of life for the one you care for is unswerving. As the illness progresses and death approaches, comfort becomes increasingly important, but the uncertainty that has always been there now assumes mammoth proportions as you face the countless unknowns and the mystery that surround death. You are no stranger to the unknown but this is different and, no matter how well you have prepared yourself, the occasion will be as TS Eliot said— 'unexpected when it arrives'.

The time immediately before death and the moment of death are usually the most feared and anticipated times in the whole process of caring. The many uncertainties, the degree of responsibility and the anguish associated with the occasion make this time both difficult and surreal. The responsibility of caring for your loved one as they die can be overwhelming. Their life as well as their death is literally in your hands and, although you will receive enormous support from family, friends, nurses and doctors, you are the one who will be there most of the time and the one likely to be called upon to make decisions. This is never easy and the task is that much harder if this is the first time you have been with someone who is dying and the one you are caring for is very dear to you.

This chapter is written to help you with some of the uncertainties that may arise at 'ground zero' and to throw light on the raft of changes that accompany death or herald its arrival. It deals with the physical changes immediately prior to death and the things that need to be done subsequent to it. I hope that it will help you to respond to these uncertain times, remove some of the anxiety, prepare you for what may happen and empower you to make decisions in keeping with the wishes of your loved one.

 Let it all unravel [so] it can be a path on which to travel.

MICHAEL LEUNIG

Predicting the time of death

The first thing to know about death is that it is unpredictable. It may arrive suddenly when you least expect it or, alternatively, dying may be so slow that you wonder if it will ever come. At times, death may seem imminent but for no apparent reason the person rallies, leaving you to wonder whether they are in fact dying or whether there is yet some unfinished business. This scenario may be repeated not once but several times. This unpredictable and uncertain course is emotionally draining and makes planning and organising difficult. Most family members want to be present when death occurs and so it is not unusual for them to spend extraordinary amounts of time around the bedside. If this goes on for any length of time, and death seems no closer after several days of waiting, it is quite reasonable to ask what is happening and whether you need to adjust your plans.

The best way to handle this situation is to arrange regular meetings (daily, or more often if needed) with the people involved in your loved one's care. Getting progress reports when death is near allows you to plan ahead. The person you speak to could be the doctor or the nurse and more often than not it will be someone different most days. This can create a problem as everyone, including health care professionals, interpret things differently and some of the messages may be conflicting. If this happens, it is better to point out the discrepancy as there may be a simple explanation.

Asking a doctor or nurse to try to predict the time of death will not be helpful as the prediction can only be a calculated guess based on their experience and what is happening at that moment. Getting a prognosis or estimate of how long a person may live is, according to Mal and Dianne McKissock, two of Australia's leading authorities on the subject of grief, potentially more harmful than helpful. From my experience, a prognosis distracts people from what is happening at the moment because they focus much of their attention on a time in the future that is more likely to be wrong than right. This creates anxiety that gets worse as the predicted time approaches.

This question of prognosis also arises if you or some other person has taken on the responsibility of informing others when death is approaching, particularly if these people have to take time off work and/or travel. Trying to flag death is not only impossible but puts the onus of responsibility on your shoulders, a responsibility you can do without at this time. By all means, pass on information but the decision when to leave work or to travel can only be made by the individuals themselves. It may be helpful to know that airlines will make every effort to get relatives on the first available flight and will sometimes offer fares at a reduced rate if they are told of the circumstances.

What changes indicate death is near?

The changes I am about to mention are useful markers along the dying trajectory, but remember that their absence does not mean death is still some way removed. Of the many changes that are possible, the following are the most reliable and best indicators that death is near:

- ◆ unconsciousness;
- ◆ changes in the pattern of breathing;
- ◆ changes in the circulation.

Unconsciousness

Death may be sudden and unexpected but for most it is relatively slow and follows a period of unconsciousness. The nature of unconsciousness is discussed in Chapter 6 but it is worth repeating that unconsciousness is not a state of oblivion but a form of sleep. It does not mean your loved one is unable to hear or respond. Quite the contrary, they may be drowsier than usual and this will ultimately progress to a deep sleep from which they do not awaken but, throughout most of this time, your loved one will be able to hear and their level of awareness is much greater than you could ever imagine.

Ian was a strapping 26-year-old man who had battled leukaemia for many years before his ultimate relapse. Knowing he would shortly die he asked that I keep him comfortable and refrain from any heroic measures when the time came. It was only a matter of weeks before he was admitted to the local hospital. He was unconscious from an overwhelming blood infection (septicaemia) and I duly informed the family that he had only hours to live. In keeping with our agreement, I had not commenced any lifesaving measures and arranged that he be kept comfortable.

The family was distraught, not only because he was dying but also because Ian's much loved sister would not arrive from overseas for four days. Hours and days passed and I was at a loss to explain how someone so ill could live this long. He had not stirred for four days and it was now the day his sister was due to arrive. The very moment she entered the room he opened his eyes and their eyes met. Ian smiled and sighed. He then lapsed back into an unconscious state and died later the same day.

So, yes, unconsciousness is a sign that death is near but whether it is hours or days away cannot be predicted; as we saw with Ian, there are too many unknown factors at play for us to say accurately. Our study of unconscious does, however, provide a guide. We noted that the average length of survival from the moment someone became unconscious was three days, with the shortest being one day and the longest eight. Bearing in mind what has been said about unconsciousness, use this time to talk to your dying relative, make physical contact and tell them of your movements because they take in much more than you would imagine. But try not to count the hours or days.

Breathing

It is not unusual for the pattern of breathing to change in the final hours or days of someone's life. These changes may occur in isolation but are more significant if they appear in association with other changes. Apart from rattly breathing, the changes in breathing described below may not be so significant and should be interpreted carefully in someone with pre-existing lung problems such as emphysema or those with cardiac disease.

Rapid or irregular breathing is perhaps the most commonly observed change. Breaths may be shallow or vary quite markedly in depth as well as frequency. There may be periods when breathing stops altogether for as long as 5–10 seconds (it will seem longer). The cycle of deep sighing respirations followed by progressively shallow breaths and then no breathing for a few seconds (Cheyne-Stokes respiration) is very common in the late stage of life and a relatively reliable sign that death is very near. Please note that this type of breathing can also occur in the sick and elderly who are not dying and its significance therefore depends on the context in which it appears. With both rapid and irregular breathing there is unlikely to be any associated distress and, although oxygen is often used, it is not absolutely necessary. So do not feel your loved one's care is compromised if you do not have oxygen in the home.

Sighing respirations, when each breath is accompanied by a distinct sigh, is unnerving and could indicate pain but may also result from the person's position in bed. It is a good idea to notify the nurse or doctor if this pattern of breathing appears and they will make the necessary assessment and adjustments to your relative/friend's position and treatment. Again, oxygen is not usually required.

Perhaps the most ominous of all breathing patterns is the so-called 'rattly' respiration where each breath is accompanied by an audible gurgle, once described to me by a relative as if the person is breathing underwater. The noise results from air passing through secretions that have accumulated in the back of the throat and/or the breathing tubes. As disturbing as it may sound, your relative/friend is by this stage deeply unconscious and almost certainly beyond feeling pain or distress. The fact that they do not cough when so much fluid is present in their throat serves to confirm the absence of distress. This form of breathing occurs only in those who are very close to death, so close that the breathing is labelled 'death rattles'.

Very little can be done to reduce the rattles and, while doctors and nurses know it is not distressing for the person dying, they realise this is anything but true for those present. For that reason, a significant part of the treatment is continually to remind and reassure family that their loved one has no awareness of what is happening. Repositioning sometimes helps and a drug called hyoscine may be administered in an attempt to dry the secretions, but it rarely helps. Suction is equally ineffective as most of the secretions are too far down the breathing tubes to be reached. Oxygen is frequently given but, as with all the other forms of breathing, is not essential.

Rattly respiration usually means that death is only minutes or hours away and family that wish to be present at the time of death should be notified. It is not necessary to call a doctor or nurse but most families do, if only to be reassured that all that needs to be done is being done.

Circulation

As someone edges closer to death the lips, fingers and toes often become bluish and the backs of the hands, forearms and shins develop a mottled appearance. The pulse by this time is very weak and often impossible to feel. All these signs indicate the circulation is now very sluggish and death is near. If these changes occur in association with rattly breathing, death may be only minutes away.

Bearing in mind the emphasis placed on pulse and blood pressure in the hospital situation, family may wonder why these 'vital signs' are rarely if ever checked when someone is dying. The reason is simple. Pulse and blood pressure tell us no more and often less about a situation than does a close look at the person who is dying. We also like to recognise the overall significance of death and to see it more in human than physiological terms. Dying is not a medical moment but a defining time in people's lives, and so the less interference the better.

How can someone so sick survive so long?

This is something you will ask yourself if dying is prolonged or when there is more suffering than you had anticipated. Dying can be slow, with no measurable change from one day to the next. There may be times when you wonder if your loved one is really dying, whether medication is prolonging the dying or there is some unfinished business that is keeping them alive. You will find it hard to conceive how anyone so sick can continue to live, particularly if they are not eating and drinking. You may also be physically and emotionally exhausted and, as much as you love and will miss the one who is dying, you may think it is time for them to go and for their suffering to end. Ultimately, you become caught in an impasse where part of you hopes death will come soon but another part dreads the very thought.

These questions and yearnings are not harsh nor do they reflect unfavourably on you. It is not heartless to want your loved one's suffering to end nor to consider your life without them. My impression is that most carers, relatives and friends engage in this silent discourse but, believing it to be dis-passionate, they keep it to themselves and suffer in silence. Talking about the impasse puts you in touch with what's within your heart, releases some of the emotional charge held there and dissipates some of the grief.

The final act of dying is thought to involve some form of letting go—letting go of the people and all the things that are loved and, ultimately, letting go of life. The act of letting go can be much harder for some than for others. There may be any number of fears or unfinished business, or the dying person may need some form of affirmation from those they love or reassurance that it is okay to die. Unfinished business may involve saying goodbye to someone, as with Ian, or surviving to partake of a special event, as was the case with Pam (see Chapter 6). So, if someone's death seems to be going on longer than usual, consider these possibilities and do whatever needs be done to address them. Let the dying person know if and when someone special is coming or when a significant event (e.g. birthday, anniversary) is to occur.

Giving people permission to die is a beautiful gift. To hear family say how much the person is loved, how much they have meant to their life, how much they will be missed but remembered is not unlike the loving embrace we give to a child as we settle them down to sleep. It relaxes them into letting go of fear or whatever they are holding on to. Say these things as often as you feel necessary and invite all members of the family to do likewise.

Occasionally, death may come suddenly and unexpectedly. Stories of family members leaving a sickroom to make a cup of tea only to return and find their relative has died are not uncommon. In most cases, this can be put down to the unpredictable nature of the illness but perhaps there is some connection between the two events. My belief is that there is a right time to die and, whether that death is earlier or later than anticipated, there is always a reason for it. Mostly, we are not privy to the reason but it helps our grief and erases some of the 'whys' if we can make space for this possibility. So, accepting that we do not know the hour or the day, make sure you and others say their goodbyes and share with their loved one, whether unconscious or not, everything that needs to be said. That way, if death does come unexpectedly you will not be left with that dreaded thought 'If only I had said...'.

What can you do as death approaches?

This is a difficult time for you and your family and, apart from ensuring your dying relative/friend is comfortable, be gentle with yourself, recognise your needs and the needs of those close to you, particularly children. Get as much rest as your body demands. You may not want to leave the room or the house but time to sleep, catch your breath, walk in nature or sit quietly on your own can be restorative and help you overcome the bumps along the way. If you and your family decide to do a round-the-clock vigil, I strongly recommend this be done on a roster basis to ensure the load is divided equally and that each has enough rest and/or time away to recuperate.

By now all medication given by mouth will have ceased and only that essential for comfort will be administered by injection under the skin or by means of a syringe driver. This usually includes morphine or some other analgesic, an antiemetic if nausea has been a problem and a sedative. Morphine is continued because pain does not disappear just because someone is dying. The use of sedation can be a vexed question but is often given in combination with morphine to ensure comfort. Oxygen is required only if breathing has been or is a problem.

The syringe driver is a battery-driven device that delivers the day's medication from a syringe into the tissue beneath the skin via a very fine 'butterfly' needle (a thin plastic tube). This is a safe and effective way of administering necessary medications that can no longer be taken by mouth.

As pain may arise from being in one position for too long it is advisable to turn your relative from one side to another about every four hours during the day and less frequently at night. Always ensure their arms and legs are well positioned and cushions are placed between bony prominences and the surface they rest upon. Rubbing the back, lower spine and limbs after repositioning may not only soothe discomfort but is another means of making intimate contact.

Your loved one will have stopped eating well before this but the mouth needs to be kept moist. If incontinence pads are in place these should be changed when wet or soiled. Again, you may be surprised at the amount of urine someone can pass when they are dying. If a urinary catheter is in place, the volume of urine will diminish over time and the urine will become concentrated (darker in colour). It is most unlikely bowels will open or need to open but, if restlessness does occur, constipation is one of many possible problems that needs to be excluded. Regular bed baths are necessary to maintain cleanliness, comfort and dignity. They are usually done by the visiting nurse(s) but if you prefer to do it they would be very happy to show you how. Alternatively, you can do it together. Don't take on any more than you can physically or emotionally cope with, but this form of contact may be a cathartic way for you to communicate with and honour your loved one.

Continue to clean and dress all skin wounds daily or as often as is required and change the bed linen and pyjamas to maintain dignity and hygiene. Within reason, do what you can to keep the room free of flies and insects as these can be more than a mere irritation to someone who is unconscious or too weak to fan them away.

Ensure you have the phone numbers of all key people and keep the list in a conspicuous spot. Always check on the availability of your doctor after hours and at weekends and, if they have made themselves available, add their home or mobile phone number to the list. When death is near, it is advisable to speak to the doctor before each weekend to fill them in on the situation and to ensure they will be around. If the doctor is unavailable at these times but is linked to an after-hours or emergency medical service, get the number(s) and ask the doctor to inform the service of the situation. If they are unavailable and are not linked to an after-hours service, you will need to get the name and number of a doctor or service who will visit in times of emergency or death.

How will I know when death occurs?

This may seem an unusual question but it is very relevant if you have no formal nursing training and are caring for your loved one at home alone. From a medical and legal perspective a person is dead when breathing stops and no heartbeat is audible with a stethoscope. You will know your relative has died by the absence of breathing. It sounds simple but may not be for any number of reasons.

◆ Breathing may have been so shallow immediately before death it is hard to know when it stops.

◆ Some people continue to take tiny gasps of air even though effective breathing has ceased. This gasping may go on for many minutes.

◆ You may be too tired and/or upset to make the assessment.

◆ If your vision is poor and you are alone it may be difficult to see if breathing has stopped.

Some hours after death the body becomes cold and stiff and some areas, such as the elbows, heels, feet and fingers, develop a bluish or purple discolouration. These are normal after-death changes.

Whatever the situation, just remember you do not have to make a decision or act immediately. If you think your relative or friend has died but are not certain, just sit there with your hand on their chest until it becomes clear that breathing has stopped. Alternatively, if you are too upset or feel unable to do this, call for help. If you are alone, ring a friend or relative. You could also ring the doctor or nurse if you prefer.

What should I do immediately after my loved one has died?

This is a very special moment. Sit by your loved one and spend whatever time you need to take in the situation and to say goodbye. You may offer a prayer, light a candle, place some flowers on or beside the body or perform a ritual in keeping with your cultural or spiritual beliefs. Short readings from a book or text such as the Bible or the Koran recognise the significance of the occasion and may offer solace to those present at the time. I have found selected readings from *The Prophet* (see Bibliography) both appropriate and meaningful.

It is okay to touch, kiss and cuddle the person just as it is to speak to them. When you are ready, ring the doctor or nurse. If death occurs in the early hours of the morning, you can defer phoning for many hours either for your sake or their convenience. Do what you are most comfortable with.

Do not ring for an ambulance and do not ring 000. Either of these calls could result in the ambulance officers instituting CPR and other resuscitative procedures unless there is clear documentation to the contrary. Any form of resuscitation would be futile and a most undignified way for your loved one to end their life.

At some convenient time, ensure the following tasks have been attended to.

◆ Turn off any oxygen and remove the mask or prongs.
◆ Lay the body flat with one pillow under the head.
◆ Remove all blankets.
◆ Turn off any electric blanket and room heating.
◆ Remember to phone the doctor and nurse.

What happens after a person dies?

After you have phoned the doctor and nurse several things follow. The doctor will confirm death has occurred and will complete the necessary death and cremation (if required) certificates. These procedures are necessary before the body can be removed. The certificate(s) are given to the funeral director when they come to collect your loved one's body. Copies of the death certificate are only available through the Registry of Births, Deaths and Marriages in your state or territory (see Appendix) and will be required to claim on life insurance or superannuation policies or to settle other financial or property transactions. For further information on death certificates, see Chapter 11, Practical matters to ponder.

The nurses will remove any piece of medical equipment attached to your relative, such as syringe driver, butterfly needles or catheters, and will then wash the body. You may, if you wish, do this yourself or help the nurses. As difficult as this may seem, it is a form of ritual that may ultimately help with your grieving.

After the wash, your relative will be dressed in fresh nightwear or attire that you and/or your loved one may have chosen before the death. I always encourage families to choose clothes that in some way identify the person and to do the dressing themselves. Many a time I have sat in a nearby room as this was being done and, in almost all cases, heard crying and laughter as family reminisce about the person and events that made them choose that attire. The ritual is cathartic and every family that did it was pleased they had done so. The type and range of clothing and accessories never ceased to amaze me. It has included scuba diving gear, golf attire (including shoes and putter), torn jeans, Hawaiian shirts, hiking boots, jogging shoes, favourite pyjamas, bright lipstick and expensive perfumes.

The funeral director should be notified about the death and a time negotiated for them to come to remove the body. By law the body has to be removed within eight hours of the funeral director being notified of the death. How long the person's body remains at home depends very much on your wishes but this could be affected by climate and conditions.

The time between death and when the funeral director comes is precious and may be used to say goodbye once again and to support each other emotionally. Depending on your beliefs and customs, it may also be a time for further prayer and ritual or a time to reflect on the life of the deceased person.

Saying goodbye can be surprisingly difficult. Numbness, exhaustion and disbelief can overtake you at this time and if you are in the room with others you may be a little reticent to say publicly what you feel. I recommend that each family member and close friend spend a little time on their own with the person who has died to say goodbye and share with them anything they may wish to say. This can be an emotional time but it is one that you will treasure for many years to come.

Are you certain they are dead?

There are many reasons why people ask this question. The commonest one is sheer disbelief. Even though death has been expected for some time it seems so unreal when it finally occurs that family member after family member asks the same question as if to make sure it is not a dream. Some also need to be absolutely certain their relative/friend is dead for fear they may wake up alone in a strange place. If this concerns you, make sure you ask for confirmation—not because that type of thing happens, but if not checked and double-checked the possibility could haunt you over the following days. The absence of breathing and a heartbeat is an absolutely sure sign that death has occurred and your doctor will make certain of this before completing the necessary certification.

Confirmation of death is also taken as permission to grieve openly and to express emotions that may have been held in check during the last days of the illness. It is thus a release, but also a surreal realisation that the person has died and that your life will be forever different. CS Lewis describes it as like losing a leg—part of you has been taken away.

Should we involve the children?

How should children be told? Should they see the dead person? Should they attend the funeral/cremation? There is no simple answer to any of these questions. Circumstances surrounding the death, family beliefs, customs, the children's ages, their relationship to the person who has died and their wishes will all influence the final choice. Because the matter is so complex it is better to have thought about these questions well before death when you were in a clearer frame of mind. Addressing the issues early also ensures the children are involved and aware of what is happening and gives them opportunities to ask questions and talk about how they feel. It also allows you to speak to a counsellor or social worker if the circumstances are particularly difficult, as with the death of a parent, or if the child seems extremely distressed or, alternatively, unaffected, neither of which is abnormal.

When a child is told about a death it is preferable that this be done by someone very close to them and in a place where they feel safe enough to cry and express their emotions. Inform the child clearly and directly about what has happened. Don't be afraid to use the word 'dead' or 'death'. Euphemisms should be avoided, as these only create confusion in the mind of the child. Give them sufficient time to take in what you have said and to ask questions. Don't be misled by a prolonged silence, or the absence of tears.

Children's responses are totally unpredictable and may range from an apparent lack of interest to aggressive behaviour. Don't misinterpret this, as it may be the only way the child can show their grief. Depending on the response, cuddle them or give them space but most importantly give them time. Then and only then, ask them if they would like to accompany you to say goodbye to the dead person. Again, give them time to ponder their answer. If it happens to be 'no', check with them a little later to make sure they have not changed their mind. If they say 'yes', prepare them gently for what they will see and what they may like to say. Then, hand in hand, lead them slowly into the room, halting if they seem to baulk, reassuring them you will go slowly and that there is no rush. Once there, give them whatever time they need but watch the non-verbal cues closely. Generally, children cope much better with death than we give them credit for.

Whether children should attend the funeral/cremation will depend on many of the factors outlined above. Providing the children are old enough and there are no unusual circumstances, my habit has been to encourage families to let the children decide. When it comes to grief, children often take their cues from the adults and, if you consider it natural and normal for them to attend, so will they. Children may feel overlooked if they are excluded from this ritual. To be looked after by friends or neighbours when they know other family members are attending the funeral can be very unsettling and leave them with many unanswered questions.

**We can make our lives sublime
And, departing, leave behind us
Footprints on the sands of time.**

HW Longfellow

8 Care of a child

It is loving that saves us, not loss that destroys us.

GEORGE VAILLANT

*t*his chapter looks at the wide-ranging problems that invariably arise when a child or adolescent is dying. This tragic situation is now, fortunately, much less common in western countries than it once was. In the early part of the twentieth century every family could expect one or more of their children to die but now, in developed countries at least, the number of infants under the age of one year that dies is extremely small. Unfortunately, the same cannot be said for children of indigenous people, poorer nations and developing countries where infant mortality remains unacceptably high and the death of a child before teenage years is relatively common.

Paediatric palliative care specialist Dr John Collins, writing in *Death and Dying in Australia*, said that in 1997 throughout Australia there were 1341 deaths of infants below the age of one year and 726 deaths of children aged between 1 and 14 years of age. This is a remarkable turnaround from 100 years ago. Similar improvements have been recorded in most developing countries and, while this is a reassuring trend, it is small consolation for parents whose child has died or for those watching helplessly as their child is dying. If anything, it adds to a parent's grief, knowing their child is one of a very small number that die each year.

Given these numbers, there are relatively few doctors, nurses or other professional people with much experience in the care of dying children—I have cared for only a handful over the last 35 years. The death of our daughter, however, taught me more than I could ever have gleaned as a doctor, and much of what I have to say comes from that one experience.

In this chapter I also raise the special needs of children when someone close, whether sibling, parent or grandparent, dies. These situations are more frequently encountered than the death of a child and, depending on who it is that dies and the circumstances of the death, it could be the most traumatic event a child is ever likely to face, with emotional and behavioural repercussions that go on for years. On this matter I draw heavily on other people's experience as my involvement with bereaved children, although frequent, is often limited to days or weeks before the death and for a brief period after. As you can imagine, many of the issues arise well after this time when, as with adults, the reality of the loss hits home.

The dying child

In all but the very young, children with a life-threatening illness do have some insight into their situation and the concept they form of their illness and their fate is pieced together from many experiences. Unremitting symptoms, frequent tests, hospitalisations, the effects of treatment, the sight of others like them and their ever contracting world convince them that something is not right. This, together with the messages they receive, the behaviour of others towards them and the observation that their life has not only changed but that it is different from that of their siblings and friends, leads them to conclude that all is not as it should be.

How and when this progresses to an appreciation of death and the knowledge that they are indeed dying is impossible to know. Children, like adults, live in the hope that what they go through in the name of treatment will make things right.

They suffer all this, not only hoping they will improve but often to satisfy doctors and family who reinforce the need for treatment for exactly the same reason. To see your child suffer is extremely traumatic but the alternative, death, is almost more than any parent can endure.

Kids are very astute and when things are not going well they pick up the subtle body language just as well if not better than adults. At some deep level they become aware of their fate even though it may not have been conveyed to them in words. Like adults, they frequently know more than they say. Dr Elisabeth Kübler-Ross spent a lot of time working with children who were dying of cancer. Many of these children had not been told about their illness or that they were dying. Almost all, however, were aware (that they were dying) and, while many lacked the verbal skills and/or the opportunity to communicate specifically about their illness, they depicted it accurately and vividly in drawings or play. One of the drawings done by a young child with an undisclosed brain tumour featured a large 'lump' on the side of his head. This communicated to all that he knew about his tumour. Not only did he have this awareness—the drawing localised the tumour to its exact position and other parts of the drawing gave a clear indication that he knew he was dying.

What death means to any child is little short of guesswork. Many hypotheses exist but they are only guides and do not tell us what it is like for any individual child. This is, of course, equally true for adults. Children don't have a well formulated view about death—in fact, for them it often has a nebulous or foreign meaning. On the other hand, they do have a lot of unanswered questions that they are often afraid to ask or do not know how to ask. Even though they may not understand, most appreciate that death results in some form of separation from those they love and, like adults, their fear is of the unknown. What Philippe Ariés said of adults is equally true for kids (perhaps even more so): 'Adults are afraid of death, as children are afraid of the dark.' This analogy not only helps us understand how children perceive death but also how you as a parent can best help them confront the unknown.

Neva
The last child I cared for was a young girl aged five years who had been sick for much of her short life. Neva's life revolved around hospitals, tests and treatments and all of that must have been as frightening to her as any dark lonely night. Her parents accompanied her through all of it and their presence no doubt gave her the courage to face the 'dark'. When treatment was no longer effective and the endless round of visits to the doctor, tests and treatment had ceased, attempts were made to prepare her for her inevitable death. While I was not present as that delicate matter was explored, I visited her many times after and during those visits it became clear that death for her meant separation from those she loved, and what she feared most was the thought of being all alone in a dark coffin. This was enormously painful for the parents to hear and for any five-year-old to bear, particularly as she had rarely been alone at any time in her life.

How do you talk to a dying child?

There will be no shortage of advice about how to talk to your child about illness and death. Everyone has an opinion and these opinions, even those of the so-called experts, are often conflicting and frequently add to your confusion. By all means, listen to what the experts have to say but trust your own intuition and think twice about doing something that does not feel right. The relationship between a child and a parent is as unique as it is special and your child will seek to recapture as much of this as possible during times of illness. With all the changes that illness brings, one of the few things that remains stable and gives a certain security is your love and the relationship that has formed over the years.

What your child needs most throughout their illness is your presence and your love. You may at times feel overwhelmed by all that is happening or unsure how to respond to difficult situations or probing questions. As threatening as these may be, do not ignore them or dismiss them. You may not know what to say or how to say it, and you may not be able to make things better, but remember that nine-tenths of communication is non-verbal and so it is the quality of your relationship and not what you say that matters. Given this, the following pieces of information, gathered from a variety of experts, may be helpful.

As a parent, your focus in dealing with your sick child is always to try to make things better. You relieve pain, soothe aches, and provide nourishment for the body and nurturing for the soul. You do whatever you can and often go to extraordinary lengths to ensure your child's needs are met. With the prospect of death there is little else you can do but, with Dylan Thomas, 'silently rage, rage against the dying of the light'. Death is not a problem that can be solved and in the case of a young child it is an outcome that we all dread and hope never to face. To have your child predecease you is confronting and painful. According to an ancient Chinese legend, the greatest blessing that can be bestowed on any family is to have the oldest die first and for no child to predecease their parent.

The difficulty you face or have already faced is the move from trying to solve problems to just listening. In his book *Care of the Soul*, Thomas Moore puts this in perspective when he says:

> The basic intention in any caring, physical or psychological, is to alleviate suffering. But in relation to the symptom [problem] itself, observation means first of all listening and looking carefully at what is being revealed in the suffering.

We are referring to your child's suffering and you being there for them, but the same is also true for you. To have someone who can do for you as you do for your child is a blessing for which you will be eternally grateful.

So how do you comfort a child in the shadow of death? In his book on *Death, Grief and Mourning*, John Stephenson quotes the wonderful work of Myra Bluebond-Langer who points out the loneliness of dying children as they try to protect their parents, while the parents at the same time 'defend their child against the awful truth'. Such collusion serves only to isolate one from the other—the child dies with both parties knowing this will happen yet unable to share their deepest feelings, which become more painful the more they are locked away.

 We feel loneliness only when we run from it.

ROLLO MAY

Running from our fears not only intensifies our loneliness but also that of our child. This running may take on forms other than avoidance. It can be disguised in futile attempts to solve all the problems or by efforts to make things better. Thomas Moore urges us just to be there, to be honest and as vulnerable as the situation demands ('just' does not imply this is easy). Allowing a child to determine the course of a conversation often results in prolonged and painful silences. These are not vacuums where nothing happens, but quite the opposite. They are the times when children search for what is in your heart and mind and may ask a profound question or make some revealing comment. So:

♦ Allow your child to determine the pace and content of the communication.

♦ Avoid meetings set up for the sole purpose of talking about death. This often results in more rather than less pain for all concerned.

♦ Do not enter into any conversation with a set agenda, remembering that an agenda to heal only gets in the way of seeing.

◆ The topic of death may or may not come up. If it does, allow your child to explore their own concept of death but answer all relevant questions honestly and as openly as possible.

◆ Do not be afraid to show emotion as this may free your child to do likewise; it lets them know, rather than suspect, what it means for you. Children and teenagers understand the language of emotions better than words.

◆ If you talk about or show your pain, remember to reassure your child that they are not responsible and you do not hold them to blame.

◆ Tell them how much you love them and how much they mean to you.

◆ If your child raises real concerns or fears, explore realistic ways of dealing with them. The young girl, Neva, that I spoke of earlier in this chapter was not frightened about death per se but by separation and the thought of her (her body) being all alone in a dark enclosed coffin. This was an equally painful thing for her parents to hear but, among tears and much angst, they explored this and other fears. What started out as a dreaded subject became the catalyst for a moving and healing dialogue between parents and child.

◆ Give whatever time is necessary for dialogue, but ensure wherever possible that time and space is made for the 'normal' things in a child's life. Like any adult, kids with a life-threatening illness oscillate between a world of sickness (with the fear of death) and one of relative normality. When they are into the normal things of life they do not need to be reminded of death. There will always be plenty of time for that.

◆ Uncharacteristic behaviour and/or emotional outbursts all have a root cause. They are often a cry for help.

◆ Make time for and be aware of the needs of other children in the family.

- ◆ Make sure the school and the parents of your child's best friends know what is happening. These friends are often pivotal in your child's support network and frequently seek and need support from their own parents, teachers or school counsellors.

 The difficulty lies not in solving problems but in expressing them.

TEILHARD DE CHARDIN

How should pain be treated?

It goes without saying that a child's physical comfort is maintained to the best of our ability throughout the course of their illness. Children may not complain, even when pain or other symptoms are present. They may have difficulty describing how they feel and, when they do, it can be hard for someone else to appreciate the level of their discomfort. Physical pain may manifest as a behavioural problem, restlessness, difficulty with sleeping or emotional withdrawal. The younger the child the more real these difficulties become. Adults who are dying frequently underplay their symptoms and carers, including doctors, underestimate their complaints. There is every reason to believe the same is true, possibly more so, with children. This being the case, we should give them the benefit of any doubt and consider a trial of treatment or increased doses of treatment if we suspect a problem.

The question of treatment is far from simple. Not only do we have the problem of assessing symptoms, there is also the added concern that no parent wants their child to have 'drugs' if they are not absolutely necessary. Such a dilemma can only be worked through by discussing the pros and cons with your own doctor. I would generally recommend a trial of treatment if there is any doubt. If the drug happens to be morphine, all the myths and misconceptions about its safety and dangers come to the surface. What was said in Chapter 3 about morphine and the adult patient is equally true for a child. If morphine is being considered this may be a good time to review that information before a final decision on treatment is made.

Should we persevere with food?

The question of food and fluids for children is no different from that for adults. Give them what they want and only when they want it. Fluids help to keep the mouth and throat moist, reducing discomfort and lessening the risk of throat infections. Fluids of any type will suffice, so be guided by your child's fancies. Ice blocks do the job perfectly well and are often considered a bit of a treat. At this stage in your child's illness, appetite may be poor and food may make them feel less well than they are already. Make the offer by all means but do not be surprised if they say no. If they do want food, give them what they want in small amounts—the sight of a large serving may be enough to turn them off eating. Psychologically, it is better that they ask for more rather than struggle with and leave a larger serve partly eaten.

Intravenous or subcutaneous fluids are rarely indicated even when your child stops eating or drinking. Fluids given in this way have no nutritional or life-sustaining value and may result in unwanted side effects. Children with a life-threatening illness do not die of starvation or dehydration but from the effects of their disease. They do not feel hungry and, if they do feel thirsty, the only way this can be eased is by keeping the mouth and lips moist.

Do deathbed visions (DBVs) or near death experiences (NDEs) occur with children?

Many people, including the Australian researcher Cherie Sutherland, have examined this question. Her work clearly shows that children do have NDEs and that they are very similar to those experienced by adults (see Chapter 6, States of consciousness). Because of the similarities between NDEs and DBVs it is reasonable to assume the latter also occur. The younger the child, however, the more difficult it may be for them to communicate their experience.

> Neva often slept with her parents in their generous king-size bed. One morning, as her father got up to make a cup of tea, he noticed Neva seemingly wide awake but with her eyes fixed on an open window. He was quite surprised when she did not respond to his morning greeting, and that her gaze remained unbroken as he walked through her field of vision. She looked so peaceful he decided not to disturb her, and went into the kitchen. When he returned a few minutes later and went to greet Neva, he was shocked to find she had died. Her death was not unexpected but the timing surprised him. Only minutes before she had appeared more awake and peaceful than for some time
>
> Days later when Neva's father was reflecting on this event, he said it appeared as if Neva was staring at something. He was not aware of anything unusual other than her fixed gaze and her apparent serenity. She appeared to be looking at something, but what, we will never know. Neva did not talk a lot about her dying but I suspect she knew death was imminent. Late in her illness she asked her family to care for her much loved puppy and to make sure it was registered. I was there at the time and this request had all the hallmarks of unfinished business.

 **This bird
longs to fly home
too long the night
which keeps her prisoner.
Eyes strain now
waiting for dawn's light
to beckon her away
from the cage she knows so well.**

See her now
watching—restless
gently fluttering
longing for the skies.
The window in her heart opens
she is mesmerised
by the rays of light
she'll soar into forever.

ALIA KAZAN, *Sitting at the Edge of Two Worlds*

Your grief

Throughout this chapter I have referred to the enormous grief
parents feel when one of their children is dying. There must
be very few life events that have such a profound and long-
lasting effect as the death of a child. The only thing I have
seen that exceeded this was the devastation of a young couple
who lost two children within the space of 18 months from
SIDS (cot death).

Your grief starts the moment you first suspect or become
aware of your child's illness. From that time on, news about
your child's progress, all the tests and treatments and the
amount of pain influence the nature and intensity of your
grief, just as the length of the illness, the amount of suffering
and the nature of the death will in the future. The flavour of
your grief is also a result of things happening inside you and it
is this that makes your grief unique. The importance of this
lies in the realisation that you cannot compare your grief or
measure your progress against others; if two of you are grieving
it is very likely you will be in different 'spaces' for much of the
time. This can put strains on the best of relationships and, if
the uniqueness of grief is not appreciated, unrealistic
expectations and added tensions will surely arise.

If other children are involved they too grieve for the loss of
their brother or sister and, like you, they also grieve for the

loss of security and stability that existed beforehand. More than ever they need your love and reassuring presence.

 The task a person can and must set for himself or herself is not to feel secure but to be able to tolerate insecurity.

ERIC FROMM

Can anything be done to help me in my grief?

There will be days when you feel life is not worth living and you cannot bear to face another day. This is not unexpected or unusual and, while it may be hard to believe now, this blackness will ultimately lift. The pain of your loss will always be there but you and your way of life will return to a semblance of normality at some unpredictable time in the future. Anniversaries and other reminders will always provoke feelings of sadness and loss but over time the wounds will heal. Grief does not like to be contained and there is plenty of evidence to suggest that those who express their grief fare much better physically and psychologically than those who do not show or talk about the way they feel. The finer points about living with grief are covered in the next two chapters but a few things are worth repeating now.

As grief starts from the moment your child's diagnosis is made, and sometimes before, whatever you can do from that moment on is helpful. That may involve unburdening yourself with your spouse/partner and/or best friends, and finding space outside the 'sickroom' that you can escape to when the need arises. What you do is a matter for you to decide but the important thing is to do something and not to be inhibited by a sense of obligation or feelings of guilt. This may not be appropriate if death is imminent or during times of crisis but, if the illness is chronic, then time to yourself can help you as well as the quality of the relationship with your child, partner and other children. You need to give yourself permission to do this—if you don't, who will?

If I don't take care of myself who else will?

ROLLO MAY

Communication is often the means used to solve problems but with grief there is no solution. The purpose of communication in your situation is not to solve problems but for you to unburden yourself. It involves telling others how you feel and knowing those people hear what you say. You may feel terrible in the process but the release is a safety valve for emotions that would otherwise build up and possibly explode. Being a two-way process, it also helps the other person(s) appreciate a little of how you feel.

The position is reversed when your sick child, spouse/partner or other children talk to you. This can be painful and difficult at the best of times but is worse when you are intimately involved with what is happening and have hardly enough emotional reserve for yourself, let alone those who are unburdening. You can usually sense whether this is a crucial time, a time to stop and attend, but if you are unsure give them the benefit of the doubt. 'Intuition is the voice of the soul,' says Gary Zukau and, if we listen to it, it rarely lets us down.

Say everything that needs to be said

After your child dies there will always be the inevitable regrets but the ones that hurt the most are thoughts about things you wanted to say but didn't. Opportunities to do this cannot be made, they just happen; and they usually happen at the most surprising times, like the middle of the night or during a wash, and following a prolonged silence. The things you and your child may wish to say can only happen if the environment is right—not just the physical environment but the emotional and spiritual climate. Your task is to continually create an environment where this can happen and, if it does, that is wonderful. If it doesn't, then what you have created may have been sufficient for your child to know what is within your heart. The language of intuition is the native tongue of any child.

Children have great intuitive sense and if they are not too sick they will ask the important questions at just the right time. But, be prepared, as the question may be blunt or somewhat obtuse. It is a matter of tuning into their wavelength, being absolutely honest and specific with your answers and avoiding as much as possible the use of euphemisms. When it comes to an understanding of death children are no more and no less wiser than adults, but they do know when we are being evasive. If you don't know the answer, say so, and throw the question back, asking what your child thinks. What starts off as an innocuous inquiry may develop into a deep and meaningful dialogue. What children often seek is an opportunity to talk rather than an answer to their question.

 One does not set out to solve problems but to create an environment where problems are resolved.

ANON

Honouring your child's life and death

Death may be forbidding and frightening but the time immediately before and after provides opportunities for you to honour your child. These opportunities will not ease the pain but they may free you from some of the helplessness that prevails. The thought of honouring someone around the time of their death is not new and in times past this took the form of rituals. Unfortunately, rituals have all but disappeared from western society and those that remain run the risk of becoming mere formalities. This is in stark contrast to 'less' developed and eastern countries which maintain rich traditions and rituals around death.

Here are a few things you might like to consider.

◆ Do what you possibly can to ensure your child dies 'well'. That may include a pain-free death and dying at home—if that is not possible, ensure the hospital/hospice environment is as you and your child would want.

◆ Do what you can to ensure your child does not die alone. This is something you cannot achieve on your own. You will need to enlist the support of others. Despite all the best laid plans your child may still die just at that moment when no one is present. This can be devastating, particularly if you have done everything to assure otherwise. I like to think there is a reason for this happening and I believe that, in some strange way, it is a child's final gift to the family. This is something only you can interpret and understand.

◆ Plan some form of ritual for when your child dies. This may take the form of readings, stories, music or song. Partake in the washing and the laying out that follow death and invite other members of the family to be part of this (if they so choose). Dress your child in their favourite clothes and put a favourite toy/item beside or on their body.

◆ Light a candle and keep your child at home for as long as you choose, remembering eight hours is the supposed maximum stated by law.

◆ Plan a burial or cremation that celebrates their life and acknowledge openly how they have enriched your life.

Further down the track you may find a cause you wish to pursue that is in some way related to your child's death. This is by no means the norm but for some it becomes another way of finding meaning in what has happened. After our daughter died of SIDS my wife and I became active members of the SIDS Association, and for some years acted as the local support people for others who had a cot death. Another person whose son was killed in a motor vehicle accident lobbied hard and long, but successfully, to have certain police procedures changed. All these things may seem insignificant, yet they are important; in some small way they put meaning back into life, which death otherwise threatens to remove completely.

 Everything you do in life is insignificant yet it is important that you do it.

MAHATMA GANDHI

How can I be there for my other children?

Depending on their age, children have varying levels of appreciation as to what is happening with their sick sibling. They may be unaware of the details of the illness or that their sibling is dying but, as a general rule, you should assume they know more than appearances and behaviour would otherwise suggest. If they do know their sibling is dying, their concept of death is unlikely to be as you would imagine. Depending on their age it could be either non-existent, rather simplistic like a sleep, or a frightening figure that takes people away (and can therefore 'get' them too). Alternatively, they may have an adult concept where death means the end of life as they know it.

What children do know is that things have changed within the home. There may be many more visitors, parents may spend less time with them and more with their sick sibling (or whoever is sick). They also note but fail to understand why their parents who were once happy and playful are now sad and cry a lot, and they wonder if they are responsible. There may be less time for the usual outings, stories and games. Noise and laughter that once flooded the house are now strangely absent. Meal times are different, TV is no longer banned and the phone never stops ringing. Everything around them is very different, but the reason is what intrigues and concerns them.

Kids do not welcome this type of change and will attempt to maintain or restore what has been normal for them. They will want to play and may use games to draw you back into their life. If this fails they may resort to attention-seeking behaviour. Drs John Collins and John Stephenson both say: 'Children often resort to games to keep control of their life but also to regain some control over yours.' They may also become surprisingly good, not only to get your attention but as a way of protecting and looking after you. Adolescents may rebel and resort to forms of behaviour that can be as destructive to them as they are disturbing to you. Overwhelming grief is nearly always behind these angry verbal or behavioural outbursts. As hard as it may be, allowing them to express these emotions even when they are directed at you is more beneficial than any reprimand. This is painful stuff and professional guidance is often required to help you navigate such a difficult course.

These scenarios are hard to avoid as the repercussions of illness and death spread far beyond the visible horizon and may engulf many innocent people in their wake. The loss of what was once normal, the uncertainty and insecurity that follow are all part of a child's grief and cannot be avoided. To the best of their ability, children need to understand what is happening to their sibling and why their own life and relationships have changed. This does not alter their grief for what is lost, but it may remove the sense of abandonment and guilt that invariably goes with it. It is not uncommon for children to wonder if they are to blame for whatever is happening or, alternatively, they may blame their sick sibling. Either scenario will sooner or later result in guilt.

There are no rules to follow but the siblings of a dying child need to understand and be understood. In keeping with what has been said about grief to date, let them ask the questions and if for any reason they cannot, ask them how they feel or how things have changed and take your cues from there. Young children may not understand when you ask how they feel. In that situation it is okay to ask if they feel sad. Give them plenty of time to think and reflect and be as vulnerable as they are. There can never be too many cuddles and kisses!

All that has just been said is also true, to a greater or lesser degree, when death involves some other family member. Grief associated with the death of a parent equals, and generally surpasses, that associated with the death of a sibling. The role the person played in the life of the child and the circumstances surrounding the loss are the two most important factors that influence a child's grief. Death of a parent not only results in the loss of a very significant person but also the object of the child's love and affection. This results in ongoing and seemingly insurmountable changes that the child must contend with. Given the shock, disbelief, devastation and loss of control that accompanies such tragedies, it is not surprising to know that the death of a significant person can be more difficult for children than for adults and that emotional, behavioural and social difficulties often ensue.

The task for the surviving parent(s) is monumental as they struggle with their own grief while attempting to give emotional and physical support to the child (children) and keep the home together and household running. There is no easy answer to this dilemma but I like what Richard Lamerton has to say—'Don't try to be too wonderful, let others help.'

9 The inner journey

People die the way they live.

ANON

*e*ach of us is a unique and special person. Our personality is the visible manifestation of a complex dynamic, the part of us that others get to know, like or dislike. We have a genetic form that is moulded by life's experiences and directed by our personal, cultural, religious and spiritual beliefs. But there is also a subconscious and an unconscious that we barely get to know. The perception of who we really are is, not surprisingly, anything but clear to ourselves, let alone others. This is not only because of the subtle effects of the 'invisible' unconscious but also because we, for a number of reasons, only reveal those parts of ourselves we are happy for others to know. The impression other people form is equally distorted by the spectacles through which they view us 'as they fail to see because of the pictures they paint on the glass' (Anon).

Rarely do we reveal that which is precious, singularly important or too painful to talk about. Sometimes, these matters are so deeply buried they are not accessible to the conscious mind but nonetheless exist. The time of death is one of the few occasions when deep or concealed matters can rise to the surface and influence the way a dying person feels and behaves. This can result in familiar but somewhat exaggerated behaviour, or behaviour that is quite out of character. Behaviour may also be the product of an internal conflict where a person struggles with the decision to reveal or conceal something of importance.

Reconciling such a difference is always liberating, particularly for those confronted by death. I do not wish to imply that every dying person has a skeleton in the cupboard or that the skeleton, if it exists, needs to be dealt with. Far from it; such an attitude would be counterproductive to any form of healing that might otherwise occur. Significant issues, however, do frequently arise and, when they do, it is important to allow the person to talk rather than for us to seek to reassure or solve the problem. Being fully present and listening with an open heart and a closed mouth is all that is required; any form of disclosure could be cathartic and healing in its own right.

If a dying person starts to reveal their innermost secrets or emotions, you may feel inadequate to deal with the situation. This is not an abnormal response. If it should happen, take a deep breath, cast aside (as best you can) your own fears and anxieties and trust yourself and the occasion. The dying person is speaking to you as their spouse, partner or friend. They are not expecting you to solve their problem, offer reassurance or venture forth with some hastily formed advice. Be reassured by the fact that the dying person has chosen you to receive their innermost truths and know that they want nothing more than your time and undivided attention.

 Nothing can be more useful to a man/woman than a determination not to be hurried.

HENRI THOREAU

The inner journey of a dying person is as individual for them as their personality. The adage that people die the way they live is a good piece of wisdom that can help us understand the journey they make as they edge closer to death. If someone has been angry throughout life, don't be surprised if they are angry around the time of death. Similarly, someone who has always cared for others may be more concerned about the welfare of the family than their own predicament. So, the more you get to know someone in life the more you will understand them, their needs, wants and fears as they die. I learnt this lesson very early in my palliative care career and, as is often the case, my teacher was one of my patients. His name was Sam.

Sam was an elderly man who had reluctantly agreed to his landlady's request to enter the hospice. I will never forget our first meeting. He was unshaven and unclean and clearly uncomfortable with the spotless hospice surrounds. His hand was bandaged and as the dressing was removed he winced but never complained. Half of the hand had been eaten away by cancer and a large gaping hole was present where his armpit should have been. I was amazed that any person could have let things get to this stage, knowing how painful it must have been.

The cancer may have been beyond cure but I knew something could be done to ease Sam's suffering. To my surprise he refused my offer of pain relief and the more I pressed the more adamant Sam was in refusing it. Finally, he said, 'I want to get out of here'. I had overstepped an invisible boundary. He insisted on leaving but as it was then late in the day he agreed to delay his departure until the morning, on the proviso there would be no further mention of pain relief. I breathed a sigh of relief and left, wondering what had gone wrong.

I rang the landlady to inform her of Sam's decision. She was not surprised and told me all she knew about Sam. He had spent all but the last few months of his life as a vagrant, sleeping outdoors, usually on park benches. He was a loner, his own master and never once sought or received help. I immediately understood why he was so uncomfortable with me, my plans for pain relief, and the surrounds he had unhappily found himself in.

I entered Sam's room the next morning, half expecting him to have vanished overnight. He was still there, propped up in bed, picking over a breakfast with his one good hand. I apologised for yesterday's events and attempted to say goodbye. Sam said, 'I'm still going but need my trousers cleaned.' He pointed to the drawer and sure enough the trousers were dirty but more in need of a resurrection than a clean. I said they might not be ready until tomorrow. 'That's okay', was Sam's reply. The next day I returned with the trousers. 'Thanks, but I might stay another night,' he said. And so he did. In fact, he stayed until he died some weeks later, having had no pain relief or any other medication throughout his whole stay.

Sam taught me that people do, indeed, die the way they live. Their ability to do so, however, is often influenced by the circumstances they find themselves in and the degree of support they receive. Sam had little of value in life other than life itself and the freedom to make his own decisions. The cancer was robbing him of the former and I, with my talk of pain relief, was robbing him of the latter. Once we got to know Sam, things changed and he was able to negotiate his illness and death in a manner of his choosing. Sam was anything but ordinary. Some may describe him as a misfit, but aren't we all? Being a misfit is nothing less than being unique and it is in our uniqueness that we find dignity in life and in death. Much of our life is spent searching to understand and have others accept our uniqueness. When our inner and outer world is in harmony with this aspiration, life flows and obstacles that once appeared insurmountable become unimportant. Such congruence is even more important with death and forms the basis of Rainer Maria Rilke's exhortation 'Oh Lord, give each of us his own death.'

Things do not always work out as well as they did with Sam, or that's how it may seem on the surface. Many times I have left a dying person's side, feeling I had let them down in their time of need, only to hear at some later date how much they had benefited from the meeting. So often it is our own sense of inadequacy and helplessness that colours the end result. Dying people do not seek answers but they do seek opportunities for expression. Never underestimate the power of two vulnerable people making meaningful contact. The words do not seem to matter, as care is not measured by what you say or do but by how prepared you are to listen. Richard Kalish's twist on a well known saying tells us how it is done— 'Don't just do something, sit there.'

A final word of caution: the assertion that people die the way they live is generally true and a good indicator of how each of us might behave when threatened by death. The danger is that this adage, if applied strictly, may see individuals labelled and packaged because of their past—other aspects of their nature that may have rarely surfaced but nonetheless exist could be easily overlooked because of a preconceived idea. When death threatens, change follows, so remain receptive at all times to the potential for change, not only with your loved one but also with yourself and others.

Grief

The process of change, the emotional ups and downs and the existential crises that occur when someone is dying are all parts of a grief reaction. The Oxford Dictionary defines grief as a time of intense sorrow and sadness, and indeed it is, but it is much more than that. Grief is a whole-body experience and not just an emotional reaction. It occurs in response to loss of any form. In the context of dying, this involves countless losses, not the least being the impending loss of one's own life. For you, the carer, relative or friend, it involves the loss of someone you love and loss of a way of life.

Grief manifests in many ways and its expression depends as much on the individual as on the situation. It is as unpredictable as life itself and the intensity of grief can vary enormously over any 24-hour period. The emotional component may be powerful and overt and, if so, grief is easily recognised. If, however, grief takes on some of the other guises mentioned in the box below it can be overlooked. In the case of a dying person, the symptoms may be wrongly attributed to the underlying illness.

THE MANY FACETS OF GRIEF

- **Physical**. *Loss of appetite, intense fatigue, difficulties with sleeping, constipation or diarrhoea, palpitations, sweating.*
- **Mental**. *Apathy, forgetfulness, difficulty in concentrating.*
- **Social**. *Withdrawal from friends and relatives; lack of interest in family and local activities.*
- **Psychological**. *A wide range of emotions of varying intensity and duration. These emotions often come in waves, reflecting the natural ebb and flow of despair and hope.*
- **Existential**. *Questioning the meaning of life and death as well as religious and spiritual beliefs.*
- **Paranormal**. *Unusual experiences are not uncommon when someone is confronted by the prospect of death. More is said about this in Chapter 6, States of Consciousness.*

Grief is a normal response to loss and, in the context of dying, may be profound or prolonged. Grief does not follow any pattern and the grieving process is as individual as personality, so do not be alarmed if the descriptions that follow do not accurately describe what you see or feel. Grief arises from issues deep within and, just as a mirror reflects only superficial features, emotions and other visible features of grief are poor images of what is happening at a much deeper level.

Grief brings forth a whole raft of changes, not only for the one who is dying but also for family and close friends, and the resulting dynamics may be as distressing as the thought of death itself. One person I cared for recently said her greatest concern was not that she was dying but that her dying was tearing her family apart at a time when she longed for closeness and intimacy. While she struggled with the reality of approaching death, her family retreated from their own pain and sense of helplessness by distancing themselves physically and emotionally from the situation. There was no question about the love they felt for each other. Grief, however, had driven a wedge between them and rendered them as strangers, lost to each other at the time of their greatest need. It is so easy to become lost in our own grief and in struggling to keep our head above water we can become blinded to what is happening around us.

Dr Elisabeth Kübler-Ross was one of the first doctors to popularise the notion of grief in the context of dying. Current opinion suggests that her views may not be entirely accurate but they have contributed greatly to our understanding of the subject. She believed that grief occurred as a result of actual or anticipated loss. Grief, she said, is a whole-body experience and, while emotions take centre stage, the physical and mental effects and the ramifications of these on our life are as real and often as crippling. She described how grief unfolds and, while this was considered gospel for many years, her initial description has since been reviewed and reshaped. Grief does not necessarily progress in recognisable stages. It is often unpredictable and as changeable as the weather but, like the weather, there are features and patterns we can recognise.

I spend the remainder of this chapter talking about the different emotions that, together with other changes, combine to form the grief response. To describe each emotion separately, as I do, is artificial and potentially misleading— emotional states rarely exist as pure entities but as a kaleidoscope of feelings that has the potential to change with every turn in a person's life. It does, however, help us to appreciate the many 'primary' emotions that mingle and contribute to the state of being we call grief.

What follows is based on observation and experience and is not meant to be a critical analysis of the subject of grief. It may not conform exactly to what the experts say, but my hope is that the recollections speak more about the human side of grief.

Fear

> **Fear does not stop death, it stops life.**
>
> ELISABETH KÜBLER-ROSS and DAVID KESSLER, *Life Lessons*

Professor John Hinton in his classic text, *Dying*, lists many emotions that are aroused by the prospect of death but says that fear is the commonest. Fear characteristically varies in intensity throughout an illness. Some days it may be overwhelming and crippling, throwing a dark and lengthy shadow over life. At other times it may be almost non-existent. The reason for these fluctuations is not always clear; external factors may account for some of the changes but they may also be due to a survival mechanism where the psyche temporarily dissociates from what is really happening. Such dissociation is not uncommon and is a healthy coping mechanism, offering periods of respite for all concerned. Don't be surprised if fear reigns supreme one day and is gone the next.

A dying person's fear may have a specific focus—fear of death, fear of suffering, separation from loved ones or being alone at the time of their death. It may also be existential, as the dying person questions long-held religious or philosophical beliefs or the meaning of life. Mostly, it is a fear of the unknown.

Fear of death is often replaced by the fear of how the person will die, when it will happen and whether suffering will be part of that final act. The fear of death is never lost but rather seen as inevitable and accepted only because there is no escaping it. If there is no escape, they are more likely to focus attention on what is equally frightening but potentially within their control. In this case, it is often the manner of dying. In my experience, most people, particularly those with cancer, expect that they will die in pain. Those with lung cancer or emphysema are particularly concerned about the possibility of choking or suffocating in some way.

Sometimes, the dying person's fears are more akin to worries and relate to practical issues such as how their spouse/partner will manage or who will care for children. They may also be consumed by financial matters (more common with men), outstanding or unfinished household repairs, a car, a pet, their prized collection(s). Such concerns may seem trivial but if they are raised they are obviously important.

Whatever the fear or concern, no matter how significant or seemingly trivial, the opportunity for the dying person to talk and have someone listen is most therapeutic. A resolution may be possible, particularly if the problem is of a practical nature, but for all matters the opportunity to unburden can in itself be therapeutic. If the fear is overwhelming, persistent or difficult to talk about, the assistance of a qualified counsellor may be necessary. Your general practitioner is the best person to advise you on these more complicated situations.

Depression

Depression may not be something a dying person complains of, or is even aware of, but it is present in a large proportion of those who are dying. It is frequently overlooked, as the cardinal symptoms and signs of depression are sometimes indistinguishable from those of the underlying disease. Sadness, loss of appetite, lack of energy, loss of interest and difficulty sleeping are common to both depression and advanced disease and it can be difficult to know which is responsible. The simplest way of determining whether a person is depressed is to ask the obvious question—do you feel depressed?

Depression is a very normal response to the ravages of illness and the associated losses the person has suffered or is likely to suffer. The medical and social consequences of a terminal illness are 'painful' enough. Add to these the fear of the future, of suffering, of dying (or of not being able to die), concern about being a burden to the family and separation from all that a person loves, and it is not surprising that depression should occur. What is more surprising is that depression is not seen in everyone who is dying and depression does not always turn into despair.

The difference between depression and despair (pathological depression) is subtle and one can imperceptibly merge into the other. While hard to make, the distinction is important. Despair is a much more serious form of depression, more disabling, associated with morbid thoughts of death and suicide, and frequently improves with antidepressant medication. There is no single feature that helps to distinguish one from the other, but the feelings of hopelessness, sadness and remorse are generally worse and talk of suicide more common in those with despair. The desire to die is not pathological and may in fact be normal in the circumstances. On the other hand, a slow death or a belief that they cannot die may be more of a worry and more likely to lead to despair.

In my experience, one of the main features of 'normal' depression and what distinguishes it from despair is the retention of some purpose or meaning in life despite all that is happening to them and around them. This purpose often revolves around family and long established relationships, the need to complete some unfinished business or the hope of surviving until some special person arrives or a significant occasion is reached. This hope of survival not only gives the terminally ill a purpose in life—when attained it also gives them permission to die. So often we see people die a short time after their last wish has been fulfilled. Several stories appear in the book that illustrate this point.

One of the best ways you can care for someone who is depressed is to create a space where they feel safe and secure enough to talk. They may not use the word 'depression' and they may find it difficult to talk about how they feel, but they will be able to talk about their losses and other important things. Issues that may also arise include how the illness has affected their life and relationships, the things they are now unable to do and what death will rob them of. Be careful, however, not to make this a question and answer session. Allow the person to talk, let them direct the flow of the conversation, but listen carefully for cues and follow up with statements like 'Tell me more about…'.

Such talk may be accompanied by tears. This can be disconcerting and the natural tendency is to change the subject in the belief it is too painful for the person to continue. Nothing is further from the truth. Tears suggest you are talking about issues that really matter and this ultimately brings healing. There may be more reason for concern about the person who never cries.

In the face of tears it is best to remain silent and, if it seems appropriate, to make some physical contact to show that you really hear their pain. This contact must be appropriate—a hug if you are family, or a simple holding of the hand. Remember, the contact is not made to stem the flow of words or outpouring of emotion; if it does, withdraw a little and ask them to continue.

During these times you too may be brought to tears. This is not only normal but, in showing your vulnerability, you demonstrate your humanness and compassion. This becomes a catalyst for the dying person to continue with whatever it was that brought on the tears. A word of caution, however: if your response is extreme or you are inconsolable, the focus may shift from the dying person to you. The outpouring may cease, not only now but also in the future, for fear of upsetting you again. If you are unable to contain your emotions or you find the going difficult, seek a friend or counsellor to talk to. This will give you an opportunity to let off steam and provide a safe and supportive environment to explore your own feelings.

I should remind you that your relative or friend, although dying, is still very much alive. Don't feel that life and death issues must be raised every time you talk. There is so much in their life to remind them of death, the last thing they need is for others to constantly remind them of the fact. People remain who they are even in the face of death and in the absence of pathological depression will continue to enjoy and seek normal conversation as they did before their illness. Some days they will want to talk of life and living, what is happening in the world, share a yarn or even tell a joke; at other times they may be more reflective and wish to talk about their illness and dying. Your task is to tune in, read their mind and body language and go with whatever is happening at that moment.

As the illness progresses and death nears, people's staying power diminishes and their interest in the world and things around them contracts. They may talk less and their ability to speak of the real issues diminishes. At these times, silence and non-verbal contact become more important. Sitting in silence for prolonged periods is often more meaningful than the spoken word. Little sharing may take place but the dying person needs your comforting presence and love as much as ever. Silence is a powerful means of communicating not only between people but also with oneself. More is said about this in Chapter 7, What happens around the time of death?

Guilt

Guilt may arise over almost any issue. Those who are dying may blame themselves for the pain and suffering of others, for the 'trouble' they are causing, for 'abandoning' their family, for not having provided for them as well as they would have liked or for failing to complete a long-promised job. They may also blame themselves for falling ill or for not responding to treatment. These regrets are normal. Unreal as they may be, the dying person needs to talk about them if only to dismiss them.

Occasionally, their thoughts may become anchored on some unhappy and, until now, long-forgotten event. This may be a quite trivial past hurt or a wasted opportunity, but sometimes it can be more painful and invoke shame as well as guilt. There is a reluctance to talk about anything that involves guilt, but when shame accompanies guilt the reluctance and the need to talk are usually much greater. Unburdening may then assume confessional proportions as the person seeks forgiveness as well as understanding. They may struggle for weeks to let go of the thing that troubles them. Ultimately, and only with enormous courage and unending trust, they seize the occasion and reveal all. This is often followed by a profound silence and enormous relief, which may be expressed in tears or a hug.

 The split between the way a person feels on the inside and the way she appears on the outside is usually maintained at considerable cost, with increased feelings of meaninglessness and decreased feelings of choice.

STEPHANIE DOWRICK, *Intimacy and Solitude*

Henri Thoreau said 'the mass of people lead lives of quiet desperation'. Maybe he was right, and, if so, I wonder how many die with years of guilt locked inside. Mick could easily have been one of these except for one precious moment.

Mick was in his late forties, of Eastern European background. He had come to Australia 15 years earlier. He was a loner, had few friends and his only remaining family lived overseas. He was admitted to the hospice with a diagnosis of end-stage AIDS and at the time his major complaint was constipation. Well, that is what the referring letter said but, when asked, Mick's response was 'I am full of shit'. I was taken aback by his descriptive language but assumed this meant he was indeed constipated.

Mick proved to be a real challenge. He was a very angry man and frequently abused the staff. Despite his manner I persisted in my efforts to befriend him and did everything possible to fix his 'constipation'. Each day I would ask Mick 'how things were' and always got the same reply—'I am full of shit'.

In time I realised that Mick was not constipated. So, when I next visited, I pulled up a chair, sat beside him and said, 'Mick, tell me what you mean when you say you are full of shit.' A long silence followed. I knew something was happening and, although tempted to ask again, I remained silent. All of a sudden Mick started to sob and managed to blurt out, 'I am full of shit because I raped my younger sister before I left home.' I was stunned and did not know what to say. Silence reigned as he continued to cry. I stayed with him for quite a while and, although few words were said, there was no lack of communication. Mick had, at long last, openly acknowledged his shame and freed himself from the terrible guilt that had plagued him for the past 15 years. Whether he was able to forgive himself I will never know, but he died several weeks later a much less troubled man.

I tell this true story not because such events are common but to show the importance of trust in a caring relationship. Dying is a very scary business but trust and meaningful human contact give people the courage to share their good and not so good life experiences.

This element of trust is like gold for a dying person. They need to trust that the doctors, nurses and carers know what they are doing and will guide them through this frightening and, for them, unexplored territory. They depend on the support and encouragement of their family and friends. They need to trust these people to journey with them as far as circumstances allow. They know that they alone must make the final transition but are comforted by the knowledge they will not be abandoned irrespective of what happens, what is said or how long the dying takes.

The opposite of being in despair is believing.

S. KIERKEGAARD

Hope

That well known saying 'Hope springs eternal' says a lot about the value of hope and how we depend on it during difficult times. Realistic hope is a catalyst for living. Unrealistic hope, on the other hand, leads us, as if blindfolded, down a dead-end street. The longer we travel this road the harder it is and the less time we have to retrace our steps and find the right path. Contrary to popular belief, hiding the truth rather than telling it is what undermines hope. Awareness of the truth inevitably leads to a re-evaluation of life and a reassessment of hopes. In the context of illness, it may lead to the hope for cure being replaced by 'mini-hopes' such as the hope to remain pain-free and independent and to live as long as possible. The transition is not easy, but failing to make the shift and living in a state of denial is ultimately more harmful.

Bob was transferred to the hospice following treatment for a brain tumour. The transferring letter said he was unaware of the diagnosis as his wife and two adult children had insisted he not be told. I found it hard to believe that he was not at least suspicious that all was not well. He had a large scar on one side of his head and radiotherapy had resulted in hair loss. Despite my uneasiness, I agreed to respect their personal and cultural values on the understanding I would not be bound by this promise if Bob asked me directly about his condition. Reluctantly, they agreed.

For a week Bob and his family lived out this charade. Then one day as I sat beside him he asked me to tell him why he was in 'this place'. I was both alarmed and relieved. I suggested his wife and family should be present to hear what I had to say. He rang them immediately. They rushed to the hospice and within one hour of his request we were all sitting down together. His wife sat as far away from her husband as the room allowed. The two children sat by their father as if ready to comfort him. His brother was also present.

I asked Bob to repeat his question. As I carefully and slowly explained the situation, Bob took hold of his children's hands and sought his wife's eyes across the room. She was unable to engage him. I said all that needed to be said. A tense silence followed and Bob then began to cry. At this point, his wife let go with all the firepower she could muster, blaming me for his distress. In the middle of this Bob got up from his chair, sat beside his wife and spoke quietly to her. They held each other and, as they sobbed, their two children joined them and together they poured out their feelings. A few days later Bob was discharged home but was readmitted and died several months later.

Some time after Bob's death I received a phone call from his brother. He told me that, following that fateful meeting, Bob had used the remaining time to deal with unfinished family matters. He told the family how much he loved them and did what he could to ensure that his wife, who had been unwell, would be adequately cared for after he died. My confirming what he had already suspected had freed Bob to do the things he considered important in his life. He fulfilled his mini-hopes.

As a palliative care doctor I am often asked by the family not to tell their loved one that they are dying. Their reasons vary: while they may be steeped in tradition they are more often based on the belief that it would be too upsetting for the person to know. My experience has been the complete opposite. When I tell them they are dying I only confirm what they already suspect, and there is a sense of relief associated with the news. Sure, it is not what they hoped to hear but it is better than living with uncertainty. There are times when truth telling is better done in little steps than one large leap. As with Bob, the news is best given with all the family present. Invariably, it is the dying person who copes best of all.

Dying is a journey and, if someone with a life-threatening illness is unaware they are dying, they are unable to complete many of the preparatory tasks. They may be denied the opportunity to plan their future, ensure they have completed all unfinished business, say goodbye, have a say in how and where they wish to die and how they wish to be cared for after death. In other words, they could rightly feel cheated.

Life is a constant search for truth. Human nature grows rather than shrinks from its effects even when the truth is painful. We have an amazing capacity to incorporate the truth. The potential harm that arises when we hide from it or when it is concealed cannot be stressed too highly. Leo Tolstoy's classic, *The Death of Ivan Ilyich*, is a dramatic example of the destruction that may occur when truth is avoided. Never underestimate the strength and courage that we possess to overcome adversity, even when this involves death. Man, says Tolstoy 'has wings to lift him above the abyss'.

George had cancer of the throat and was admitted to the hospice with a severe chest infection. He knew his cancer was incurable but no one had actually told him he was dying. He was devastated when he heard this news but in reality it came as no surprise. He had wondered why he felt so unwell. Now he knew. Like all of us, George did not want to die. He still had a lot of living to do. When asked if there were any things he hoped for, he spoke of his only daughter's forthcoming wedding and how important it was for him to attend. Hope for cure and long-term survival had vanished but George wanted, more than anything, to see his daughter married. No guarantees were given but a promise was made to try to make this happen. Not only did George get to the wedding, he got up from his wheelchair and walked his daughter down the aisle. George completed his most important unfinished business and died shortly after.

Denial

Denial is a very useful means of cushioning the effect of any shock. We resort to it frequently in life so it is not surprising to find it very much 'alive' in the context of a life-threatening illness. Denial reliably appears when we first receive a diagnosis of cancer or some other serious illness. While it may take many forms the following statements are good examples of denial in action: 'This can't be true'; 'I will get another opinion'; 'This can't be me they are talking about'. Following the initial shock, reality ultimately sinks in and the diagnosis is acknowledged even if not fully accepted. A mixture of hope, denial and despair characterises the treatment phase of any illness, and the way we feel is influenced by the presence or absence of symptoms, the results of tests and the messages (verbal and non-verbal) communicated by the medical profession.

When treatment fails and the person is told what they fear most—'The cancer has come back' or 'The illness has not responded to treatment'— shock returns and is followed by any number of emotional responses, particularly depression, anger, fear, resignation or any combination of these. Denial may return but it is now diluted by constant reminders and visible signs such as loss of appetite, loss of weight, altered body image, worsening fatigue and numerous other symptoms.

The determination to fight the illness, the wish to survive, fear of death and a touch of denial may at this stage drive someone to look for a cure no matter what the cost. People seek out diets, complementary treatments, meditation, prayer or 'healing' of any form. Some people go to extraordinary lengths and may travel overseas or resort to unproven and questionable treatments that drain them physically and financially. Sadly, this drive to find a cure may be under the direction of a family member whose own determination may stem from their denial as much as from their suffering. Worse still, it may not be what the sick person wants but goes along with for their own reasons.

If asked about complementary therapies, my attitude is to respect a sick person's wish to explore options. I accept that these treatments may not influence the course of the illness but the measure of control they give and the ensuing journey may be more important than the outcome. The benefits of complementary therapy often appear in unexpected ways. The person may or may not feel better, disease progression may or may not slow, death may or may not be delayed. We hope for the best but, if the best does not eventuate, the sick person and their family are more likely to accept the inevitability of death knowing that everything has been tried. Because doctors do not always see the hidden value of such a journey and because they tend to look at results and outcomes, they are not always the best people to ask when deciding on the merit of complementary treatment. More information on complementary therapies appears under the heading of 'Cancer Cures' in Chapter 5, Day-to-day care.

Judy was a young woman with a rare and aggressive form of cancer found during her first and only pregnancy. Because of the pregnancy she could not begin treatment until after the delivery, by which time the cancer had spread. Not surprisingly, treatment failed to slow the growth and Judy became more debilitated and eventually required oxygen for prolonged periods. She tried very hard to be a mother to her now three-year-old son but the limitations imposed on her by the cancer made it very difficult.

She announced she was going overseas to see a healer who, at the time, had been much in the news. I was alarmed not only by the belief that it would be a fruitless exercise but also because it would take her away from her family for several weeks. I also had some concern for her safety during the travel. Nonetheless, Judy embarked on this journey and to everyone's surprise the whole trip went rather smoothly. On her return, however, she was no better and in almost constant need of oxygen.

As her breathlessness worsened, Judy found it increasingly difficult to manage at home and she was ultimately admitted to the hospice. During her stay I gathered enough courage to ask her about the overseas trip and whether she felt it was worthwhile. To my surprise she said, unhesitatingly and most sincerely, that it was the best thing she had done. I struggled to understand the meaning of her words and somewhat naively probed how could this be so when she was not cured. She looked at me and with a rather wry smile said, 'I did not go to be cured, only to be healed.'

Before Judy died I came to understand what she meant. She accepted the inevitability of her death but she could not accept, and grieved over, the fact that she would lose her son, her husband and family. She also had other important unfinished business and, as a result of the pilgrimage, had not only dealt with all these matters but had found a peace in dying that she had not considered possible before the visit. Initially, I had thought she was denying her illness but I now know it was I who was denying her needs.

This story raised in my mind the meaning of the word 'healing' and how there can be such a thing when one is confronted by death. We are all familiar with the meaning of the word 'cure', which is what others do to make someone better. It generally involves doctors doing something to the physical body such as curing infections, ulcers, migraine and so on. Healing, on the other hand, is what sick people do for themselves and, unlike cure, it usually involves the psychological or spiritual dimension. Therefore, someone may heal themselves yet still die.

So denial, except in its extreme form, is a relatively common and healthy way of coping with serious illness and the prospect of an early death. I regularly see it at play in my conversations with people who are dying. After talking for some time about their illness and their impending death they may raise the topic of a holiday, which in the context seems totally unrealistic. Is this denial or is it a fantasy, and does it really matter?

I would like to believe it is human nature at work, helping that person to cope with the emotional burden of their illness and giving them something to look forward to, no matter how unlikely. It is very similar to how we look forward to, plan and fantasise about a holiday and how the thought of this keeps us going even though we may be emotionally and physically exhausted by work or other commitments.

Does it matter? If a person talks about an unlikely or unrealistic holiday but at other times talks about their dying, then it does not matter. They know they are dying and fantasising about a holiday is not a serious denial but a way of coping with grief. Very few who are dying are unaware of their fate. We will all face death in our own particular way. From an outsider's point of view, the task is not to have a plan to keep the dying person on track but to allow them to find their own way. Otherwise, their dying becomes our agenda and, thinking they are lost, we invite them to join us on our wayward journey. This is unhealthy for all concerned, particularly for the one who is dying. In joining someone else's journey they abandon their way and are therefore less likely to be healed. Mary d'Apice in her book *Noon to Nightfall* sums this up very nicely when she says, 'You do not have to accept what people do but understand what leads them to it.'

Much more serious then is the form of denial that exists or is falsely propagated by others. Family or friends who claim that their loved one is looking better when they patently don't, or who insist they continue diets and complementary therapies when death is nigh, do serious harm to themselves, their loved one and others who collude with them. Similar harm follows if the medical profession consciously or unconsciously engages in its own form of denial by persevering with treatment when it is not working. Truth is ubiquitous and cannot be hidden or disguised by any form of denial. No one can hide from what is deeply felt and persevering with denial only adds to the isolation a dying person already feels. Ultimately, this proves more difficult to live with than the thought of death itself. Beverley McNamara, writing in *Death and Dying*, gives the following clear message:

> The experience of each terminally ill person depends to some extent on the resolution of uncertainties, but of course this resolution is closely linked to the nature of communication between professional hospital staff, patients, and their families.

Ours is both a death-defying and death-denying society and we tend to conceptualise death only as something that deprives us of life. This is epitomised by a comment made by Phillip Adams in *Death and Dying* where he somewhat flippantly describes death as 'a full stop to the life sentence'. What we have lost and what Phillip Adams ignores is the significance of death. Death is more than the end of life. It is what shapes and defines our life. Rather than a full stop it is more akin to the circumference of a circle. Just as the circumference forms the boundary beyond which a circle does not exist (at least in that form) and is what shapes and defines the circle, death similarly shapes and defines our life and forms the boundary between life and the unknown. Death is certainly not some insignificant spot. We are less likely to deny death when we do not deny its significance.

Anger

Anger, like all feelings, is a form of communication. It brings us a message.
ELISABETH KÜBLER-ROSS and DAVID KESSLER, *Life Lessons*

A dying person's anger is nearly always part of a grief reaction and is one of the hardest emotions for carers and relatives to deal with. It may be externalised and clearly visible, or internalised when it commonly manifests as a depressed state and is therefore easily overlooked. Factors that predispose to anger or depression include the loss of control of one's life, the loss of independence and the frustration that accompanies these and the many other losses that illness brings. It may take just one minor incident or a series of catastrophes to bring underlying anger to the surface but occasionally it remains buried and becomes depression. The factors that trigger the anger may be real or imaginary, major or minor. Typical scenarios include reaction to things unwanted or unpleasant, things that are not done the 'right' way, disappointments, excessive noise, people 'fussing', relatives who don't visit or who visit too often, excessive pain, the failure to ease pain and so on.

Even though a particular person or incident may incite the anger, anyone becomes fair game, particularly if they happen to be in the wrong place at the wrong time. The closer your links with the dying person the more likely you are to become the target of this legitimate but misdirected anger. Remember, you are rarely the source of their anger but you are the safest outlet for it.

When anger surfaces, give the person time and opportunity to 'let off steam'. In keeping with the well known saying that anger generates a lot of heat but not much light, the outburst may be cathartic, but if it does not get to the source of the problem (i.e. grief) it will be revisited on more than one occasion. Attending to the incident that caused the outburst may defuse the anger but will not address the underlying vulnerability and pain. Anger not only clouds thinking but also hides the truth, so the chance of healing is remote while it persists. This is not to say that anger is bad or destructive— it may be the only emotion that wakens the dying person to their pain and ultimately opens the door to the 'deeper messages'. So don't dampen, retaliate, rationalise or withdraw from a dying person's anger. It is a disguise for pain. Give them the space and security they need, stay with them physically and emotionally and in time the anger will give way to grief. If the situation does not improve or indeed worsens, advice should be sought from the treating doctor.

The situation may be extremely difficult for you if the anger does not resolve or is directed your way. It is hurtful to be the target for criticism, particularly when there is no basis to the assertion. You may feel unappreciated and somewhat compromised in trying to defend yourself or to respond. There is no easy answer to this dilemma as there are so many unknowns. The golden rule of listening rather than reacting is still the safest option. If outbursts are frequent, vindictive or traumatic, seek help. Defending yourself may be counter-productive but stating your pain clearly and non-judgementally, using 'I' messages (e.g. I feel hurt when you speak to me that way) may just be enough to turn things around.

There will be many times when you, too, become angry. This is more likely to happen as your loved one's health deteriorates and you assume more and more of the care. You may feel angry with your loved one for not getting better or for the demands they place on you. Tensions may arise from the lack of perceived support from family or for unrealistic expectations they may hold on treatment or prognosis. Your concern for your ailing relative/friend, your helplessness at not being able to make things right may predispose you to uncharacteristic outbursts. Tiredness caused by an ever-increasing number of demands, lack of sleep and efforts to maintain some sense of normality in your life can compromise your health and also your emotional state.

Don't hesitate to tell your loved one when you feel tired, stressed or in need of a break. This level of honesty facilitates a form of communication that encourages understanding and resolution and will circumvent crises. The need for a break is not a sign of failure. Persevering when you are physically and emotionally exhausted benefits no one and may be more harmful to the one you care for than it is to yourself. Seriously ill people are very attuned to what is happening around them and it will come as no surprise when you tell them how you feel. They know what it is like to feel exhausted and will understand your need for respite. When a need such as this conflicts with your desire, take comfort in these words:

Your soul is sometimes a battlefield, upon which your reason and your judgement wage war against your passion and your appetite.
Would that I could be the peacemaker in your soul, that I might turn the discord and the rivalry of your elements into oneness and melody.
But how shall I, unless you yourselves be also the peacemakers, nay the lovers of all your elements.

KAHLIL GIBRAN, *The Prophet*

Anger may also arise out of misunderstandings or confusion about treatment, particularly if you and your loved one get conflicting information about what should be done or when your expectations for treatment are at variance with what is happening. This is more likely when your relative is transferred from one place of care to another (e.g. home to hospice) or if there is a sudden change in their condition or when death is very close. Good and ongoing communication by way of regular meetings involving your relative/friend, family, doctors and nurses is an effective way of preventing or dealing with these problem areas. These meetings are organised as a matter of routine when someone is admitted to a hospice or palliative care unit. They usually take place several days after the person has arrived. This gives staff enough time to get to know your relative/friend and to have a better appreciation of the overall situation. There is, of course, no barrier to an earlier meeting if you feel it is necessary.

Joy

The discussion so far has been confined to a set of emotions most commonly associated with a life-threatening illness. Individually or collectively, these emotions form part of the package we call grief and, while they are no longer seen as unavoidable milestones along the way, there is an expectation that many or all of them will occur at some time during the course of the illness. This expectation may have a subtle influence on the nature of care given and the focus we maintain throughout a person's illness and their dying. As we become caught up in the gravity of the situation and our own responsibilities, we can so easily overlook priceless moments or not fully partake of the times of joy and happiness as they appear.

Pick up any book that specialises in grief or talk to any doctor about the subject and you will find the focus is almost exclusively on what, for want of a better word, I describe as 'painful' emotions. I am not suggesting that grief is not painful, but am pointing out the tendency that we all have to get caught up with the darker side of grief.

In a humorous but worrying snapshot of the medical profession, Dr Marc Cohen states that medicine is obsessed with negative rather than positive mental states. He reviewed the medical literature over the past 30 years and found that 300 000 articles have been published on pain, depression and anxiety but only a mere 3000 on pleasure, joy and happiness. This may say something about the seriousness of the work, but it also makes me wonder if this seriousness is reflected in the attitude doctors bring to their work and the expectation they have of those they treat.

One of the real hazards faced by people who are seriously ill is the risk that their disease may overrun their life and the care they receive. If care deals only with pathology, it can result in the human spirit dying well before the body succumbs. Seeing the one you love die is hard enough, but watching them change and at times become unrecognisable is also painful and can lead the family to say that the person in the bed is no longer the one they knew. Many years ago my daughter, who was eight years old at the time, said to me after an unhappy experience with an adult that the difference between adults and children is that adults forget how to have fun. Not only is this generally true, it also suggests that happiness not sadness is our natural state. Laughter comes more easily than tears, a smile is more common than a smirk, we naturally seek pleasure rather than pain and we find love more replenishing than hate. If we have a greater longing and natural capacity for positive emotions, surely this longing must be as great, if not greater, during times of grief? It is said that grief is a response to loss. Maybe joy needs to be added to the long list of losses.

What has this got to do with palliative care and, more specifically, with the care of your loved one? Simply this: do not be consumed by the occasion. Be aware of how easy it is to be caught up with caring and to neglect nurturing. Despite the responsibilities that go with caring, the pain and suffering that you and your loved one will endure and the sadness that hangs threateningly over your lives, there will be times of joy, happiness, excitement, awe and wonder. These moments do not need to be manufactured for they will appear spontaneously, as if arising from a natural spring. Quite often they arise by way of reminiscing about the funny, the bizarre or the unusual. Even things that were once painful are, in time, often seen in a more humorous light. When these moments arise embrace them, enjoy them, bathe in them and do not feel guilty for the pleasure they bring. Reminiscing is an excellent way to communicate, to bridge barriers, to contact emotions and ultimately to heal. So do not hesitate to pull out photographs or show videos as a way of creating an environment for remembering.

Dying is painful and sad for all concerned but it does not exclude humour or joy and is only made worse when we miss moments of happiness or opportunities to laugh. Tears of joy are as effective in relieving pain as are tears of sadness.

 **She who brings herself a joy
does the winged life destroy.
She who kisses the joy as it flies
lives in eternity's sunrise.**

WILLIAM BLAKE

---

10 Your journey after caring is complete

> The death of a loved one is a deep wound that heals naturally provided one does nothing to delay the healing.
>
> PHILIPPE ARIÉS

*t*wenty-six years ago our fourth child Moira died as a result of a cot death. Despite the intervening years I remember the day as if it was yesterday. It was 3 pm and I was sitting in my office dictating letters when my secretary put a call through from my wife, Ann. I don't know why but I sensed something was terribly wrong. There was a brief moment when time appeared to stand still, as if to draw my attention to what was about to follow. Then, choking on her words, Ann managed to tell me that our youngest child Moira, born just four weeks earlier, had died. Every ounce of energy drained from my body as I stared blankly at the wall ahead. There were no thoughts, no feelings, just over-whelming numbness. That moment is forever etched in my mind and memories and emotions flood back even as I write about it.

Nothing anyone could have said would have prepared Ann or me for that moment, or for what was to follow. Our lives, our relationships with each other, our children, family, friends and colleagues were turned upside down. We felt as if an invisible force had violated us. We felt threatened by the enormity of the event and helpless to know what to do. The control we usually held over our life had, in an instant, been wrested from us and we laboured through each minute of each hour of each day. Ultimately, pain replaced numbness, meaningless days followed restless nights, disturbing thoughts and unanswerable questions filled our minds and death, now unmasked, started to consume our life. We were increasingly troubled and haunted by an event we could not yet comprehend.

How you feel, behave and think following the death of someone close is unimaginable, and the experience will surprise you as much as it will pain you. There is, as NW Clerk said, 'a kind of invisible blanket between the world and you'. You not only lose someone you love but also a way of life and a way of being. Life is cut short 'like a dance cut in mid career or a flower with its head unluckily snapped off .... so many roads once; now so many culs de sac'. This is how Clerk described his own grief after the death of his much loved wife from cancer. Elizabeth Lee likens the feeling to the moment of birth where there is both agony and incredible love.

We are creatures of habit and the way we grieve is a reflection of how we have always coped with adversity. The loss of someone you love will have you retreating into all the familiar ways. If you have previously cried when you were upset, you will cry when you grieve. If anger, silence, caring for others or getting on with things was your habit, it will now be your crutch. Grief will have your signature all over it and will teach you more about yourself than most other things in life. So never question why you feel a certain way or why you do or don't do certain things. 'Why' questions are only confronting and confusing. Don't disown the feelings and behaviours or try to change them but rather get to know them and experience them. They are then more likely to open and reveal a part of you that until now may have been the silent partner in your life.

I cannot be sure of how you or anyone will grieve but the following comments reflect common responses and patterns of grief. You may recognise some part of you in there and it may throw a little light on your own grief and the journey you are now on.

What can you expect?

Grieving is a complex process and the way you grieve will be influenced by many factors, including:

◆ your relationship with the person who has died;

◆ the nature and duration of that person's illness;

◆ the coping mechanisms you usually adopt;

◆ the length of time you had to prepare for the death;

◆ the manner of the person's death and the amount of associated suffering;

◆ the suddenness of the death;

◆ any recent bereavement;

◆ religious and spiritual beliefs;

◆ your value system;

◆ your culture;

◆ other stressful situations such as life event issues and personal or relationship problems.

The way your grief unfolds and the way it will affect you are totally unpredictable, but what is certain is that the intensity of the emotions that form a large part of grief will be unlike anything you have experienced before. John O'Donohue described grief in his book, *Anam Cara*, as a journey that is only a quarter inch long and several miles deep. This is not meant to imply that the grieving period is short, rather that the depth of the emotions is profound. It also suggests, correctly, that improvement is very slow and mostly imperceptible. This 'stuckness' is what makes one day seem as bad if not worse than the last. You will frequently feel all alone as if in a deep dark hole, and wonder whether there can be any escape. Slowly, almost imperceptibly, the grief eases and you will climb out of this hole. Some sense of normality will ultimately return and the wounds begin to heal, though not completely.

This journey you must take that we call 'grief' is not out and back. You are unlikely to return to the same point at which you started. Not only does your life change but so also will you. Grief will reshape your life, your priorities, your beliefs, your attitudes and your faith. Grief induces change like nothing else you will experience. Grief takes you apart and, in putting the pieces back together, you will be different with a changed perspective on life as well as death. The repercussions of your loved one's death will be felt throughout the family, among friends, colleagues and perhaps the local community. Grief casts its net widely.

For a considerable time you will feel numb and dazed and you will function somewhat automatically. You may find yourself doing familiar things such as cooking or setting the table for two or buying food the deceased person liked to eat. You may also live in expectation that they will walk through the door at any time or be at the other end of a ringing phone. Long established routines will be lived out in your mind and the pain that accompanies these allows grief slowly to permeate the numbness. It is only when all the essential paperwork has been completed and most of your friends and relatives have returned to their respective worlds that the full impact of the death hits. It is then that you realise your loved one is not coming back.

Grief usually hits a peak four to eight weeks after the death. During this time and for many months after you will travel on a rollercoaster of emotions with many ups and downs and twists. Many of these emotions may even appear in a single 24-hour period. Reminders like a favourite tune on the radio, a photograph that you recover, mail addressed to the deceased, memories of things you did together can put you in a spin, when only moments before you felt you were coping well. Do not shirk the painful memories or reminiscing. Hiding from them does not make the pain go away or the journey any easier. It is usually better to deal with grief up-front rather than fight a continual rearguard action. The poet Rilke puts this in more symbolic terms: 'If the devils are driven away the angels will also take flight.'

How will I feel?

The duration and course of your loved one's illness will greatly influence the way you feel after they die. If there has been a lot of suffering or if the illness was prolonged, you may feel relief when death finally arrives. Relief may also be felt because the responsibility you assumed in caring for your loved one has now passed, or some unfinished business was completed before the time of death. The relative of one of my patients described this as feeling 'sadder but lighter'. There are many reasons why you may feel sad but relieved; this is absolutely normal and not an indication that you do not care.

Anger, resentment and intolerance are also very common and may be directed to the one you were caring for or to other members of the family for things they did or did not do. These emotions and any resulting conflict are almost inevitable in a caring situation and do not in any way indicate an absence of compassion or love. In fact, it is often because of love that they arise. Professor David Kissane, writing in *Death and Dying in Australia*, emphasises that feelings of resentment, conflict and love can coexist. When contradictory feelings arise, don't push them away. Acknowledge them and hold on to them in a space of love. It is the failure to recognise and own these uncomfortable feelings that causes harm. The feelings themselves are normal and often transient. It is the expectation we have of ourselves that makes them seem abnormal, keeps them alive and can make us feel guilty.

If death follows closely after diagnosis, anger and resentment may be directed to the medical profession. This may involve their failure to effect a cure, the type of treatment your loved one did or did not receive or for inadequately informing you of the seriousness of the situation. Alternatively, you may just feel angry. There may be no particular focus for your anger—you may be angry with the whole world and with your God. Whatever the reason(s), don't harbour this emotion, bring it into the open and look at it. If a person is the object of your anger, talk to them and attempt to resolve the problem with good communication. But do this only when you are not consumed by anger. Aim to achieve a win–win outcome. If anger is directed to the one who has died, talking it through with a friend or someone you feel comfortable with is helpful.

If the death involved a lifelong partner or a child it is not unusual to feel that life is not worth living. Occasionally, thoughts of suicide may be entertained. Early in my career, a reaction like that would have had me scurrying for a prescription pad or the telephone to make an urgent referral to a psychiatrist. I have since learnt that the wish not to continue living occurs in a very high proportion of those who grieve and is an expression of grief rather than a death wish. Suicidal thoughts spring from a deep sense of loss and talking about it takes courage and indicates a desire to heal the wound. The greatest risk is not with those who talk about suicide but with those who don't, or those who try to talk and are not heard. Morbid thoughts are persistent and/or intense in up to 10 per cent of the bereaved. If you have this experience I urge you to talk to someone—it may be very difficult to negotiate this course safely on your own.

Grief may also affect you in many other ways. Grief can impair your thinking and the way your body behaves. Lack of energy, aches and pains, difficulty sleeping (or excessive sleeping), loss of appetite, nausea and weight loss can often have you believing that you too are unwell. Other symptoms such as forgetfulness and an inability to concentrate may reinforce a belief that you are losing your mind.

When I was in private practice it was not uncommon for someone to visit me shortly after the death of a relative/friend with symptoms similar to those of the deceased. They feared for their own health and the convincing nature of their symptoms brought them along. More often than not these symptoms were a reflection of underlying grief, a grief that had gone unrecognised. This so-called 'somaticising' of grief occurs with both sexes but is thought to be more common among men. Men and women readily admit to physical symptoms but some will rarely talk about emotions and find it hard to believe their pain and lethargy arise from unacknowledged sadness, anger or depression.

Possible repercussions

Death or even the anticipation of death has effects that can temporarily destabilise the immediate family. Each family member grieves differently, depending on their emotional as well as their familial relationship with the dying person. This, together with the altered family dynamics, can induce tensions, put strains on relationships and alter the normal process of decision making. Occasionally, family tensions or disagreements that appear after death are the smouldering remnants of discontent that first appeared during the course of the illness. According to Andrea Sankar, many of these conflicts can be traced back to longstanding relationship difficulties that are usually kept hidden.

Changes in roles, responsibilities and expectations are inevitable both before and after the death and this remodelling of the family unit can induce its own grief. Disagreement and hurt are sometimes inevitable, but the likelihood of long-term damage is reduced if family members communicate with each other, remain tolerant of different opinions and are prepared to be flexible. You will discover there is not one single way to grieve. As indicated earlier, the course of your grief and the strategies you use will be different from those of any other person involved. There is therefore a need for tolerance. After the death of our daughter, for example, I found myself on a completely different path from Ann and for a time that proved difficult and lonely, as we were lost to each other. This dissonance is not at all uncommon, particularly with parents who have lost a child, and may result not only in emotional separation but physical separation also.

It is not unreasonable to expect a spouse, partner, close friend or relative to be the most supportive and understanding person in times of grief, but often they are not as they struggle with their own pain. If dissonance is a problem or if the risk is high, as with the death of a child, I recommend counselling early rather than later. However, I have found that individuals and parents are often reluctant to accept counselling as they see the need as a failure on their part. The opposite is true. To seek help in the face of grief is a sign of strength and indicates a desire to heal.

My own inability to cry not only surprised me but made me question my own genuineness when, as a doctor, I saw how easily others cried in the face of their grief. I could not understand how someone so overwhelmed by grief was unable to cry. Guilt overtook me as I struggled to reconcile what I felt on the inside with what showed on the outside. Ultimately, tears did come but only in the safety and privacy of our home, usually when Ann and I tried to comfort each other and make sense of what had happened. It was only then that I realised this was the way I always responded to adversity. It said nothing about what I felt on the inside. Take heed and do not make the same mistake of measuring your grief against some other person or accepted norm.

Guilt

Guilt does not need any invitation to visit. It makes regular appearances and may have top billing in any grief story. In our case, there were many 'what ifs', 'if onlys' and 'whys' that uncovered guilt and laid it out before us. We would replay the events surrounding Moira's death over and over, wondering what we had missed, what clues were overlooked and what we could have done to prevent the tragedy. As is always the case, there were no answers, just more questions and more heartache.

You too may have lingering doubts that cause you to feel guilty. These may relate to the way you cared for your loved one, negative feelings you harboured at some time towards your loved one, including the hope that death may come quickly. Caring for someone you love while they are dying is extraordinarily difficult. Mistakes will occur and emotions may at times run high but that is the norm, not the exception. I know of few if any situations where things ran without a hitch. Forgiveness, acceptance and understanding are required in large doses when you care for someone you love. You regularly shower compassion on the one who is dying and members of your own family. This is fine but you need regular servings as well. Be gentle and kind to yourself. Be very aware of your own needs and the dangers inherent in self-recrimination, as that may become a self-fulfilling prophecy.

 What a man thinks of himself, that is which determines, or rather indicates, his fate.

HENRI THOREAU

Guilt is often more subtle and may occur at the most unexpected times. I know of a man who, many months after his wife's death, felt guilty when his sadness started to lift. He thought the sadness and longing for his wife should have lasted much longer and was deeply troubled by their waning. Coping better than you expect, the first day you do not think about your deceased relative/friend, the first outing after your loved one's death, your first laugh can all be harbingers of guilt. Ultimately, you will be able to accept the coexistence of pleasure and pain without feeling guilt, but it can be a slow learning experience.

Remember
Remember me when I am gone away,
Gone far away into the silent land;
When you can no more hold me by the hand
Nor I half turn to go yet turning stay.
Remember me when no more day by day
You tell me of our future that you planned:
Only remember me; you understand
It will be late to counsel then or pray.
Yet if you should forget me for a while
And afterwards remember, do not grieve:
For if the darkness and corruption leave
A vestige of the thoughts that once I had,
Better by far you should forget and smile
Than that you should remember and be sad.

CHRISTINA ROSSETTI 1830–94

Managing your grief

There is no simple recipe for how to grieve but there is ample evidence to suggest the time course is shorter and the outcome better in those who express their emotions and talk about the way they feel. Some find this easier than others, but it may also be lack of opportunity that influences the grieving process. Those who can express their feelings and have a large and supportive family and/or group of friends obviously do better than people who tend to bottle up their emotions, and are isolated or reclusive.

There are exceptions but some people, often men, grieve by getting on with the job and sorting out all the practical problems. If you are one of these, be aware there may be times when you hit rock bottom and, if you do, no amount of busyness will lead you out of the hole. Hitting the bottom may be the only way your emotions can get the message through, imploring you to stop and take note of what is going on inside. It is a call to attention, informing you that all is not well and that you should take appropriate action.

Others think they are not coping if they cry or get angry. This could not be further from the truth. The ability to express emotions is the healthiest way to grieve. Talking about the way you feel and expressing emotions acts as a safety valve and prevents an excessive build-up of pressure. Shutting off this avenue of release can result in an unhealthy and possibly dangerous build-up that may manifest in other ways such as depression or ill health.

Two of the biggest problems I faced in my grief were lassitude and my reluctance to be with people. Clerk calls this 'the laziness of grief'. Getting up in the morning was a monumental task and the thought of facing another day was often overwhelming. Physical and emotional exhaustion never left me but it was the lack of motivation that made the most mundane of chores almost insurmountable. If and when I did get started, I was surprised to find how relatively easy most things were. Starting was the real problem. Once I appreciated this fact I set myself a manageable number of jobs to do each day. This routine gave some semblance of structure to an otherwise disorganised life, helped guide me through each day and prevented the endless jobs piling up. My lifelong habit of jogging was temporarily shelved but, when I did resume, I quickly came to appreciate how much this activity contributed to my recovery. I now recommend some form of daily exercise, preferably walking, to any grieving or depressed person. Regular exercise, particularly in a natural setting, has a profound healing effect on body and spirit. It frees the mind, allowing deeper wisdom and knowledge to break through the barriers we may have constructed to protect ourselves during times of grief.

Returning to work or resuming your 'normal' life may be

another hurdle to contend with. The physical and emotional effort this involves, or the assumption made by others that you must be 'better', can make this a difficult time. Returning to 'public' life exposes you to one of the most seemingly benign but difficult situations you are likely to encounter after your loved one's death. Responding to the questions 'How are you?' or 'How are you coping?' can be surprisingly difficult and confronting. I certainly came to dread them. I was uncertain whether it was just part of the routine social engagement or whether the inquirer really wanted to know. In my case, a truthful answer was generally ruled out because circumstances were not right or because I did not have the emotional stamina to unburden myself once again. So I learnt to dodge the question with a nod or a shrug. Eventually, I did need to confront some friends and colleagues who, through pity or genuine concern, would ask the same question several times a day as though they expected me to fall apart at any moment.

Unfortunately, grieving people are also open game for gratuitous advice. This is rarely helpful. The worst piece of advice I received was that I should return to work as soon as possible because it would help me to forget. After all these years those words still grate, and at the time they wounded me deeply. I certainly wanted to feel normal and was prepared to do whatever it took, but I did not want to forget. I had so little to remember of Moira's short life I wanted to hang onto every little thing that reminded me of her, no matter how painful. Shrouding grief with an early return to work was not going to aid my healing and is unlikely to benefit you.

Returning to 'normal' life was equally difficult for Ann. She was relatively isolated at home, but it was the isolation she felt as people crossed the street or changed direction when they saw her coming that was painful and made her feel like a modern-day leper. Fortunately, there were also those who went out of their way to be with her. The most helpful were those who listened and really heard her distress. For those who do not know what to say or are fearful of saying the wrong thing, a touch or an embrace is all that is required to show you care.

Anniversaries, birthdays, Christmas and other significant dates can reawaken grief even if the death occurred years earlier. The intensity of the emotions after such a long time may surprise you and it is often best to anticipate these occasions and decide in advance how you wish to spend the day. You may choose to be alone or alternatively have someone special with you. Whatever you do, do not ignore the meaning and significance of these special times.

Finally, choose carefully and be selective about who you talk to. Grieving people need someone who will listen rather than give advice. Those that give advice are unconsciously putting their own agenda before yours and may only add to your uncertainty and confusion. The painstaking work of grief cannot be short-circuited but talking about how you feel makes the journey less lonely. The best person to talk to is someone you trust and who is not uncomfortable if you fall apart. Protect yourself from further and unnecessary hurt by avoiding people you do not want to see or things you do not want to do.

Take care not to neglect the basic necessities of life. Sleeping patterns change and appetite is frequently reduced or lost altogether. Try to maintain your usual time of going to bed. The nights may seem long and you may feel as though you do not sleep. You may only remember the periods of restlessness but, more often than not, sleep will appear even if only in snatches. This is better than no sleep at all, and maintaining some form of routine for going to bed and rising is more likely to see you settle back into a relatively normal sleep pattern. A bedside radio, tapes or CDs can be a comfort during the long dark hours. Hot milk prior to bed may assist sleep, whereas tannin-rich teas and coffee are counter-productive, as is the long-term use of sleeping tablets.

Food may be the last thing you feel like. This may be a product of your grief or a remnant of bad eating habits cultivated while you were caring for your loved one. Food, like sleep, is essential for your body. Physical and emotional healing can be impaired by the lack of either, or both. Try to cultivate a regular pattern of three meals a day. Small servings are less likely to be rejected than large overfilled plates. Don't eat on the run and, if there are others in the house, try to sit down together. Cooking (and the associated shopping) may be one of many chores you cannot face in the early phase of your grief. Have friends cook and do other practical things for you. This not only relieves you of chores but gives others a simple and practical way of helping and being with you.

Caregiving is physically and emotionally demanding so don't be too surprised by the consequences. Exhaustion and a whole gamut of emotions will accompany you for longer than you can imagine.

How long will I grieve?

This is a question you will regularly ask of yourself, especially when times are tough or when grieving goes on longer than you had imagined. There is no answer, nor any way to predict. Living with the expectation that 'this' must end soon is normal but unhelpful and will ultimately sabotage the normal grieving process. The answer is the old but familiar story of taking one day at a time. Just as water finds its own course following a torrential downpour so too does the flow of emotion that accompanies grief; any attempt to block or redirect the flow will only lead to a greater outpouring once the levy breaks. As unlikely as it may seem at the start, life will at some time in the future take shape and a sense of normality will slowly return. This process may take months or years and, even though the wounds heal, tender scars always remain.

Those who express their grief fare better in the short and long term than those who bottle up their feelings. If you find it hard, go through old photographs, play favourite music and visit places that hold fond memories. These are good ways to release emotions that may have settled but still weigh heavily.

Grief is an uncomfortable and unpleasant state to be in but it is unavoidable if someone you love dies. Healing and moving on in life is not possible without it. Relatives and friends may not see it this way and may suggest you shake yourself out of it, try to forget, go on a holiday or return to work. Such comments often reflect their discomfort and desire to have you feeling better. Do what you choose to do and not what others say. You are extremely vulnerable at this time and can do without unhelpful suggestions. If, on the other hand, you choose to take a holiday or return to work, that is okay, but it is good to discuss this with someone you trust. Either of these plans can introduce unexpected complications.

Several weeks after Moira's death we went to stay with Ann's family in New Zealand. This removed us from the ever present memories and we were greatly assisted by the love and support we got from caring relatives. The two weeks' respite was just what we needed and we thought we were all the better for it. When we returned home we were shocked to find how quickly the grief returned. We were right back into the rawness of what we had left behind. That was a shock and we were not prepared for it.

Finally, it is suggested that any major life decisions should be delayed and not made early in the course of grief. Stability rather than change is essential at this time. Contemplate change by all means, include all those who will be most affected by the change in your discussions, but make haste slowly.

Communicating with family

Your verbal and non-verbal communication is important when other family members, particularly children, are involved. You may not be able to help each other but to isolate yourself because you are in pain, or because you do not wish to upset one another, creates gulfs in a relationship that can be misinterpreted as not caring. Your partner, spouse and children may feel sidelined by your isolation and uncertain how best to help. Just to say you feel lousy today, or that you need space or a hug, fills the gaps that can otherwise be misinterpreted. Communication is a two-way process, so remember to check how others are and give them plenty of hugs in return. They too are hurting.

Kids are extremely intuitive and can sense when things are not right. They know their life has been disrupted but, depending on their age, they may not always associate this with the death. Their confusion is further complicated by all the resulting changes within the household, the loss of security and seeing people they love cry, possibly for the first time. One of the commonest ways they manifest this confusion is through changes in behaviour. So be understanding, and give them plenty of time. Tell them how you feel and how much you love them. Explain why things are different, why familiar routines have been broken and why there are lots of visitors. Listen to their concerns, answer their questions and feel their unique form of pain. If you do not include them in your grief they may blame themselves for the way you feel and may even hold themselves responsible for the death.

Our daughters, who were aged five and three when Moira died, told us some years later they were confused by all the flurry and emotional turmoil but what disturbed them most was the sight of their parents crying. This was new to them and as frightening as Moira's death itself. They also feared her death might have been a result of something they did or didn't do. One of them was guilt-stricken and believed that putting her dirty fingers into Moira's mouth may have caused her death. Not surprisingly, she was too afraid to talk about it at the time. The lesson to be learnt is that kids can read much more into the situation and into our grief than we could ever imagine. The only way you will know this is by listening to them.

Children can move quickly between the sadness of death and the fun of childhood. They may be full of sorrow one minute but playing the next. Our five-year-old, though very sad, hoped Moira's death would not interfere with her birthday party, which had been planned for a few days later. Such ambivalence is common and very normal in children as it is in adults. Ann and I were surprised by this and many other things, but came to realise how obtuse and pervasive a child's grief can be. Our two daughters, Claire and Ruth, would cry but usually in concert with us, not simply because they were sad but, seeing both of us cry, they felt they should keep us company. Our other child, James, was almost two and, while he does not remember the occasion, I have vivid memories of him repeatedly entering Moira's room after she had died as if wondering what had become of her. His confusion was painfully obvious even if it was not stated. David was born 15 months after Moira died but even he was not immune to the effects of her death. In his early years he often asked if he was a replacement for Moira. He needed lots of love and reassurance before he was able to accept his own inherent worth.

Complicated or protracted grief

On occasions grief is complicated and protracted. This is often a result of the circumstances surrounding the death but can occasionally stem from a relationship that binds the grieving person to the one that has died and prevents them from moving on. Complicated grief has nothing to do with the intensity of emotions and problems are more likely to arise (but not always) with those who do not show emotion. Similarly, there is no time limit on how long one grieves; what is important is how grief affects a person's life and whether it becomes a barrier to their adjusting to life without the deceased.

There is no single feature that identifies complicated grief but severe or prolonged physical neglect is probably the most obvious. Refusing to eat over a considerable period of time, marked weight loss and excessive use of alcohol and/or drugs can be telltale signs. Serious mental distress, uncharacteristic or unusual behaviour, persistent morbid thoughts and disturbed thinking are more serious and may indicate a need for medical or psychological help.

The following list is not exhaustive but in the context of a life-threatening illness, indicates the type of circumstances that may predispose to protracted grief. Grief that results from or is complicated by any of these may require extra support from family and friends as well as professional help, regardless of whether any of the above warning signs are present.

- Sudden death
- Suicide
- Death in which considerable pain and suffereing is involved
- Death of a child or young person
- Death of a young mother/father
- Series of deaths
- Social isolation following the death of someone close
- Elderly person widowed after a long and happy marriage
- Financial hardship

Suicide is uncommon among those who grieve, but it is not unusual or abnormal to feel that life is not worth living or to contemplate suicide. In 35 years I have known two people who have committed suicide following the death of someone very close. Neither gave any warning despite the fact that the suicides were well planned. There were many more that I thought were at risk but who did not suicide. If you have morbid thoughts and cannot be certain of your intentions seek help from someone you trust. Ring Lifeline (see Appendix) or some other grief support service or see your doctor. This is often a difficult thing to do when you are so depressed but asking for help is the first and most important step in the process of healing. To be able to say 'I am frightened, I am scared, I am depressed' requires courage but sharing this with someone you trust, even someone anonymous such as a telephone counselling service, can be a huge relief. This unburdening and letting go of your grief is what heals.

Your concern about the emotional state of someone else who is grieving can also be a tricky situation. No one wants to overreact but neither do you want to overlook possible warning signs. If you are a close friend or relative of the person, share your concerns with them honestly and compassionately. They are unlikely to be upset by your concern and may in fact be grateful and relieved. Rather than making the situation worse, it may provide the opportunity they have been waiting for but have been too afraid to create for themselves. If you don't feel confident in doing this, discuss the situation with the person's next of kin or the family doctor.

Unusual events

One of the most common but least recognised aspects of grief is the so-called 'paranormal' phenomenon. This somewhat mysterious term refers to events or experiences that are out of the ordinary and for which there is no plausible explanation. In the context of grief these experiences may include one or more of the following:

- extremely vivid dreams in which the deceased appears and brings some form of message;
- visions of the deceased;
- the impression that the deceased is beside you;
- hearing the deceased's voice;
- a sense that you are being touched by the deceased;
- smelling her perfume or his aftershave;
- an unusual happening such as a clock stopping, a picture falling from the wall or a flickering light, just as you speak of the deceased.

These experiences are common and absolutely normal in people who are grieving. They do not mean you are going mad. The American Psychiatric Association has recognised these experiences as part of the normal grieving process. Many studies have shown that up to 40 per cent of those who grieve have at least one of these experiences within the first few months of their bereavement. Some may have many more, but this is the exception rather than the rule. The most common experience is the sense of the deceased person being present in the room, but vivid dreams or hearing the deceased's voice are also reported frequently. People say these experiences feel absolutely real and, although initially frightening, the experience becomes something they treasure.

On His Dead Wife

Methought I saw my late espoused saint
Brought to me like Alcestis from the grave,
Whom Jove's great son to her glad husband gave,
Rescued from death by force, though pale and
    faint.
Mine, as whom washed from spot of childbed
    taint
Purification in the old Law did save,
And such as yet once more I trust to have
Full sight of her in heaven without restraint,
Came vested all in white, pure as her mind.
Her face was veiled, yet to my fancied sight
Love, sweetness, goodness, in her person shined
So clear as in no face with more delight.
But O as to embrace me she inclined,
I waked, she fled, and day brought back my night.

JOHN MILTON 1608–74

I have known some relatives ask why they have not had one of these experiences when others have. Widows particularly felt a deep sense of hurt and wondered why they had missed out. We simply do not know why these experiences occur with some but not all. It is too big a question for us to understand and to suggest otherwise assumes we know what happens after death. The only reassurance I can offer is that failure to have one of these experiences often means that everything that needed to be said was said before the time of death.

The phenomenon itself has intrigued many researchers and begs the question as to whether these experiences are a form of hallucination or evidence for life after death. No proof exists either way. For me, the question of cause is academic and will never be resolved. What is important is the significance and the meaning people attach to these experiences. Although messages are rarely given, most say they 'know' what it is all about. They can describe the events quite clearly but the understanding is more of an intuitive knowing. It is something that is felt rather than heard. This may sound nebulous to the outsider but it is as real as it is indescribable for the one who has the experience.

If you have one of these experiences, treasure it and be reassured you are not going mad. You may wish to keep it to yourself but sharing it could be helpful. If you do, choose someone you trust, someone who will listen and who will validate you and what you describe.

Many years ago I was the palliative care doctor for Red. As the name suggests he had a shock of red hair which, by the time I met him, was thinning through age and ill health. He had a large cancer involving the side of his face and, despite pain and daily dressings, he did his best to maintain a normal life. This included frequent fishing holidays with his wife and three daughters, one of whom had recently married a man of Italian descent. Red loved the outdoors and, despite his rapidly growing cancer, he and his family spent their last Christmas camped on a river bank. The only thing Red loved more than fishing was his family, who in turn showered him with understanding, love and care.

During one of his hospital visits Red admitted he was not afraid of death but was worried about who would do all the repairs and practical things after he died. He had been a very practical person throughout life and this concern was real for him, as it is with many men facing the same fate. Red died several weeks after his last camping holiday. The family knew that holiday was likely to be his last so they all accompanied him for a few days while he fished his favourite spot, yarned to long-time fishing mates and said goodbye to all those familiar and treasured things.

A week after his death I was contacted by his wife who wanted to tell me about something unusual that had happened. Shortly after Red's death, her son-in-law had got up from bed in the early hours of the morning. As he walked down the hall he saw Red, as clear as day, standing in front of him. He was stunned and remained frozen to the spot. He was unsure how long the vision lasted but suspects it was brief. Nothing was said but he was absolutely certain about the message Red sought to deliver: 'You are the only man in this family. I want you to look after my wife and daughters.' The experience was so real and the message so clear his son-in-law had no doubt about its reality.

11 Practical matters to ponder

Begin with the possible;
Begin with one step.
There is always a limit,
You cannot do more than you can.
If you try to do too much,
You will do nothing.

GURDJIEFF

Caring for someone who is dying can be a difficult, time-consuming and energy-sapping business. Managing issues on a day-to-day basis is often the only way to cope and the thought of making plans for funerals or completing paperwork may be low on the priority list. If you have tried to get your loved one's affairs in order you may have found it all too surreal to continue, or the information may be hard to access or too confusing to process. I suspect that anyone in the position of carer looks for reasons not to proceed with these confronting yet necessary issues when there are so many other care-related matters that have to be attended to. Added to this are the natural concerns of how and when to raise the subject of a funeral with someone who is dying. Will it upset them and take away whatever hope they have? Is it worth the associated trauma? This is upsetting business, a series of problems you could well do without.

In this chapter I endeavour to touch on some of the issues that are best addressed before the time of death and matters that pertain to the death. Experience has shown that it is better to complete necessary business earlier rather than later, but selecting the right time will always remain a challenge. The list that follows may seem daunting but, if you begin with the easiest or most urgent task and slowly work your way through, it is not so overwhelming. Seek assistance when you need it and delegate chores if you have neither the time nor the inclination. As Gurdjieff says: 'You cannot do more than you can'!

The legal status of many of the matters discussed varies from state to state. For a more complete review, I refer you to the excellent book by Stella Tarakson (see Bibliography).

Funeral arrangements

Planning the funeral is possibly one of the most traumatic things that needs to be done when someone is dying. It could be interpreted as the final step in acknowledging the inevitability of your loved one's death and, for this reason alone, many defer making the necessary arrangements until it is too late to involve the one who is most affected. Some believe it may upset them or that it will be seen as giving up all hope. Dying people are very aware of their predicament and are not afraid of talking about funerals—they are often relieved to have the matter dealt with and out of the way. Instead of being traumatic it can be a cathartic and healing experience, providing an ideal opportunity for the dying person to reflect on their life and talk about things they have already contemplated.

A funeral is an occasion when the bereaved farewell and celebrate the life of the one who has died. It is also a statement about that person's life. If the dying person has the opportunity to plan their own funeral it can be their final gift to those who are left behind. If you believe this, as I do, the opportunity to plan our own funeral is as much a right as it is a privilege. So, put planning a funeral high on the priority list, do it while the person is able to participate actively, take plenty of time and do it in an environment suited to the occasion.

You often meet your destiny on the road you take to avoid it.

ANON

Choice of funeral director

All funeral directors stick to a code of conduct and are governed by the same rules, so the choice is usually based on practical matters such as cost and location. Reputation and other people's recommendation are sometimes useful guides. If you are unsure, visit some of the funeral directors in your vicinity before making a choice. This is one chore you could delegate to a close family member who has the time. It is a tedious task. Remember to discuss the findings with your loved one before making a final decision. Once that decision has been made, tell the funeral director of your decision, record the name and phone number and keep this with other important contacts. The next contact you have with the funeral director will be when you ring after your loved one's death.

Burial or cremation

Some people have strong views on burial and cremation while others have no particular preference. Again, it is important for your loved one to have a say but costs, circumstances, customs and beliefs will determine the ultimate choice. Information needed to assist in making this decision can be obtained from any funeral director.

Special needs

If there are special cultural or religious practices or rituals you wish to observe at and around death, ensure the information is conveyed to people that may be affected, such as nurses, doctors and funeral director. These wishes and any associated requests should be recorded and a copy given to those involved in the care of your loved one.

Keeping the body at home

There is not only a move towards people dying at home but many families ask to keep the body of their loved one at home for as long as possible after death. Current legislation allows you to keep the body at home for eight hours after death. In practice, this means the funeral director must collect the body within eight hours of being notified of the death. This arbitrary eight hours may turn out to be longer if you do not notify the funeral director immediately.

Irrespective of how long you decide to keep your deceased relative at home, remember to turn off all heating in the room, including electric blankets, and remove all warm bed covers as heat will speed up the process of decomposition. It is also important to contact the nurses promptly so they can wash and lay out the body before stiffness (rigor mortis) sets in. You may, of course, choose to do this yourself or you may feel more at ease assisting the nurses. For further information on what to do after death, see Chapter 7, What happens around the time of death.

Home viewing

A home viewing immediately prior to burial or cremation is something that can be arranged through the funeral director. It gives the family an opportunity to say a private farewell immediately before the more public funeral. Some think this is a great idea but others are concerned that the presence of a dead body in the house may create unhappy associations, particularly for younger members of the family. Again, there is an eight-hour time limit for such a viewing unless the body has been embalmed.

Post-mortem

A post-mortem is rarely required when someone's death is not unexpected and there are no suspicious circumstances. If the circumstances of death are not clear, or if the person dies within twenty-four hours of surgery or a general anaesthetic, or if a doctor has not seen the deceased during the last three months of life, the coroner must be notified by the attending doctor. A post-mortem is then obligatory. If someone has a life-threatening illness but dies suddenly or sooner than expected and none of the above stipulations apply, a post-mortem is not required by law.

Sometimes a post-mortem may be requested by the treating doctors, not out of any legal requirement but to clarify some unusual aspect of the illness. This can be a real dilemma if the request comes out of the blue and has not been discussed prior to your loved one's death. If that is the case, you should obtain as much information as possible about the reasons for the post-mortem and ask what exactly will be done and what, if any, tissues will be removed. Ask for time to think about it and particularly to discuss the matter with other family members. Ultimately, you must do what you are comfortable with, bearing in mind how your relative/friend may have felt about the procedure. If you agree to the request you will have to sign the necessary paperwork, which should include any special requests or restrictions you place on the examination. A post-mortem should not delay or interfere with the funeral arrangements and the funeral director will take the body of your loved one to and from the place where the post-mortem is to be performed.

Organ donation

Whether any of your loved one's organs will be suitable for donation depends on their age and the cause of death. Rarely are organs suitable for transplantation if the person is aged or has died of cancer or some other chronic illness. The only exception to this are the corneas (the covering over the coloured part of the eye). These can be donated irrespective of age or condition; even those with widespread cancer can donate corneas if they so choose. If your relative/friend requires further information on organ donation your doctor will advise you or put you in contact with the appropriate organisations.

Death certificate

Following the death of your loved one, a copy of the death certificate will be required to complete outstanding financial and legal matters. This cannot be supplied by your doctor and is only available from the Registry of Births, Deaths and Marriages in your state or territory (see Appendix). Applications are usually made through the funeral director. They will complete the application form and forward it, together with the doctor's death certificate and all other information required to register the death. This is done immediately after the burial or cremation. A fee of $30–40 applies, and the copy of the death certificate is usually available within three working days of application. The next of kin, the deceased's solicitor or the executor of the will can also make application by phoning or visiting the website of the appropriate registry.

Who needs to be notified after death?

Many agencies will have to be notified of your loved one's death. The funeral director can provide you with a list of the usual government contacts but there may be others. When you are speaking to your loved one about funeral arrangements, ask if there are any special friends, colleagues or associates that they would like notified after death. Some of the more important commercial agencies include:

◆ Centrelink
◆ Bank or other financial institution

- Life and other insurance companies
- Superannuation funds
- Medicare
- Roads and Traffic Authority
- Australian Taxation Office
- Electoral Office
- Credit card operators

Pensions and allowances

Illness can be a very expensive business. Medical and pharmaceutical costs pile up while financial reserves slowly evaporate. You may be one of the many people in a caring situation unaware of the financial help that is available via a carer's allowance or disability pension. If you are linked in with a palliative care service, ask to speak to their social worker. They can advise you on these and other sources of possible income, help you to complete the necessary paperwork and fast-track their processing. Alternatively, you can visit your nearest Centrelink office and discuss your situation with them.

Wills

You hardly need to be reminded of the importance of a will, but I wish to stress the value of preparing it well in advance. Like many practical issues, the matter of a will is often deferred until the very last moment for fear of upsetting the dying person. In my experience this is rarely the case—it is often something the person wishes to finalise if only to move on to other important business. It can also be a moving and meaningful experience as they decide which personal item they would like to leave to whom. Contentious issues can also arise and the earlier these are dealt with the better.

Most people have wills in place before illness becomes a reality. If the will is reasonably current and circumstances have not significantly altered there is probably no need to update. If circumstances have changed and you are concerned the will could be contested, seek legal advice. As with all things, the earlier this is done the better—the closer someone is to death the less energy and inclination they have to deal with contentious issues. Confusion is also more common as death nears and this may render the person incapable of making a legally binding will.

When confusion is present and doubt exists about the person's competence to make a legally binding will, a doctor is asked to determine their capacity to understand the nature and ramifications of the decisions to be made. The doctor also needs to be assured that all decisions are made freely and without duress. As confusion is often an intermittent or reversible problem, capacity may vary from day to day. If a person is incapable of making a legal will one day the situation should be kept under review and, if there is significant improvement, the doctor can be asked to reassess the situation.

Enduring Power of Attorney

An Enduring Power of Attorney is a legal document that gives powers to an appropriately appointed person to make and enact financial decisions on behalf of someone sick or dying. This power comes into effect only if the person making the appointment loses capacity, and it ceases at the time of their death. The advantages of having a trusted person manage financial affairs and carry out transactions in this situation is obvious. The appointment can only be made if both parties understand fully the nature of the power and what sort of things can be done. The sooner an Enduring Power of Attorney is made the better as the problem of confusion could interfere with its implementation.

Three practical points are worth noting.

1 An Enduring Power of Attorney requires a solicitor, barrister or clerk of petty sessions to explain the nature of

the appointment and to ensure all parties understand and agree with the appointment. The solicitor then witnesses the necessary completion of the certificate.

2 An Enduring Power of Attorney made in one state may not be recognised in another.

3 To act appropriately the appointed person should be familiar with the contents of the deceased's will. For this reason, it is usually the next of kin or a close relative/friend who is appointed.

Enduring Guardianship

An Enduring Guardianship is a relatively new piece of legislation that exists in some states and territories and allows for the appointment of a person to make legally binding lifestyle decisions for someone, should they lose the capacity to do so. This covers:

◆ where the person should live;

◆ what health care services they should receive;

◆ what medical and dental treatment they should receive.

As with the Power of Attorney, the Enduring Guardianship only comes into effect when the person making the appointment loses the capacity to make their own decisions, and it ceases when they die. There are restrictions as to who can be appointed as Guardian and, for obvious reasons, anyone involved directly in the medical care of the person making the appointment (e.g. doctor, nurse) is excluded. You, as carer and/or next of kin, are not excluded and would be eminently suitable to fulfil this role.

The Enduring Guardianship is a powerful and useful piece of legislation. It acts as an advanced directive, allowing the appointed Guardian to make legally binding decisions on behalf of the dying person on matters of treatment and care. It also means that doctors are unable to give treatment a

Guardian does not consent to. On the other hand, doctors may refuse to give treatment if they disagree with the Guardian's recommendation. The appointment of a Guardian is one way of ensuring that a person receives the type of care they want at and around the time of death. From a carer's point of view (subject to your being appointed Guardian), you continue to have an important and legally endorsed role in the way your loved one is treated, provided the decisions you make fulfil the directions recorded by your loved one on the Guardianship form.

Both the Enduring Power of Attorney and Enduring Guardianship are legally binding documents. They ensure that the dying person maintains control over their financial situation and the way they are cared for around the time of death. Once the documents have been completed, make sure they are accessible and available when needed.

Advanced Directive

With medical science's increasing ability to keep sick and dying people alive, many people seek to ensure that their existence will not be prolonged by treatment or technology when there is little or no hope of a meaningful recovery. Instead, they seek an assurance that they will be kept pain-free and their death will be dignified. In an attempt to guarantee this, Advanced Directives have become a popular means of stating one's wishes. Unlike Enduring Guardianships they are not legally binding and no guarantee can therefore be given that wishes recorded in this way will be honoured. As they have no legal status, they are less valuable than an Enduring Guardianship and unnecessary in states or territories where the Guardianship is valid.

Nonetheless, in states and territories where Enduring Guardianship is not available, an Advanced Directive, recently written and witnessed, is a very useful resource. Most doctors would be guided by its contents unless the requests were unusual or illegal. Like an Enduring Guardianship, it is particularly useful in the face of unexpected illness or injury, particularly where the person may be unable to give clear directions about their treatment preferences.

The Department of Health in most states and territories has available 'dying with dignity' or 'good palliative care' guidelines that may assist you in your understanding and planning of Advanced Directives or Enduring Guardianship orders. Whatever choice you make, pay detailed attention to the wording of the document, as ambiguous or vague statements can be challenged. Legal guidance is recommended and is indeed necessary with the Power of Attorney and the Guardianship.

12 Epilogue

> In gaining awareness of death we sharpen and intensify our awareness of life.
>
> H. FEIFEL

Your experience in caring for someone you love and being with them as they die brings you face to face with the reality and mystery of death. In this book I have sought to deal honestly and pragmatically with the events and emotions that accompany death but, in so doing, the mystery that surrounds such an occasion becomes inescapable. The metaphysical dimensions of death and the shifts people make as they die have been highlighted in many of the stories, raising questions for us all.

The story of Steve's final twelve months of life illustrates the potential for change and the importance of time in allowing these changes to permeate the 'excesses' that accumulate throughout life. Steve's life and death had a profound and lasting effect on me. My entrenched views and preconceived ideas were blown away during those twelve months and left me to wonder at the potential that lies within us all.

Steve was in his early thirties when he was admitted to hospital, having suddenly and for no obvious reason become paraplegic. After many tests the doctors informed him he had a rare cancer of the spine that was inoperable and also incurable. It was a death sentence, but Steve had received a fair share of body blows in his short life and he brushed it off. He greeted the news with a string of choice Australian expletives and insisted on being discharged back to his home, a single room in a large boarding house where others like him sheltered from life.

Steve was no ordinary 33-year-old. He had spent most of his adult life bouncing between boys' homes, mental institutions and jail and had moved to Sydney not to start a new life but to continue the old in a setting where he was less well known. He carried with him many labels—psychopath, schizophrenic, hard-nosed criminal, dropout, misfit. He was not a very nice person.

At the boarding house the owners did all they could to make Steve comfortable but the responsibility of caring for him in that setting was beyond them. They insisted on outside help and, despite his objections, palliative care nurses were called in to assist with his treatment and day-to-day care. The nurses were emotionally and physically strong and had successfully managed many difficult patients in the past, but they had never come across anyone like Steve. He was difficult, lacked all social graces, had a foul tongue and resisted all efforts to keep him clean. Despite this, fellow guests at the boarding house cared for him, ran his messages, placed his bets and kept him company. In return, he treated them with as much respect as he was capable of.

Out of frustration and concern for his welfare the nurses asked me to visit him. They thought he might listen to another man, a doctor and an authority figure. How wrong they were! I had done my homework and imagined how I would approach the situation. The manager of the boarding house pointed to Steve's room but then disappeared. I thought that was strange. I knocked on the door and, hearing a grunt, tentatively entered the room. Steve was stretched out in bed, naked except for a sheet covering the lower part of his body; a cigarette hung from his mouth and the bedside radio was loudly broadcasting a race meeting. I was about to introduce myself when Steve lashed out—'Who the f... are you and what the f... do you want?'

I had not expected a warm welcome but I had not anticipated this. Somewhat unconvincingly I said, 'I am

Michael, the palliative care doctor.' As I was to learn later, Steve could read a person and a situation in a flash. He knew he had the upper hand and was determined to drive home the advantage, but he also needed to check my staying power. He said, 'Can't you f...ing see I'm busy, you'll have to come back some other time.' Grateful for the opportunity to leave and take stock of the situation, I asked if the same time tomorrow would be okay. I took the audible grunt to mean 'yes' and left the room.

The next day I went back. 'It's me again,' I said, as I knocked and slowly opened the door. He was less hostile and, in between orders to people in other rooms and orders for me to open windows then close windows, he gave the impression of listening to what I had to say and he even allowed me to examine parts of his damaged body. But he remained defiant and refused to allow the nurses to do any of the things I recommended.

Several weeks passed and eventually I received the call I had been dreading. The nurses said things were getting out of hand, Steve's problems were worse and they were helpless to do anything about them. 'Could you admit him to the palliative care unit for a short time to see if that makes a difference?' I immediately had visions of Steve swearing, smoking and bossing everyone around and wondered how the staff and the other patients would cope. I tried desperately to think of alternatives but none came to mind and, after a meeting with the staff to prepare them for what could only be a torrid time, I arranged for Steve to be admitted.

My fears were well founded. Within five minutes of his admission Steve had offended most of the nurses and the cleaning and kitchen staff, as well as the unfortunate man who shared his room. Among his many orders were repeated demands that he be allowed to smoke in his room. Regulations had never stopped him in the past. After a hurried meeting with senior staff, we sat down with Steve and tried to work out some ground rules that might make life bearable for us all. He listed his demands, which included his need to smoke, place bets and have regular lashings of 'junk' food. In return we asked for cooperation with the nursing and medical care he was to receive, and at least an attempt to stop swearing. We arranged for him to be wheeled outside to a shaded area to smoke, and for volunteers and others to do his essential shopping.

The road was rocky but after one month it was clear we were making some progress. Steve hardly swore and when he did it was followed by an immediate 'Oh, s..., I'm sorry'. He and his room-mate became close friends and when the man died Steve was visibly upset and found it hard to conceal his tears.

Being a chain smoker, Steve spent more time out of his room than in. The palliative care unit had a designated outdoor smoking area. It was a nice protected spot, though it lacked a view. Tall, suffering pot plants made up for the concrete surrounds. The area was large enough to take Steve's bed and still leave ample room for other smokers to gather round. And gather they did. Steve became a popular figure with his fellow patients and also their friends and relatives. He was a great entertainer and a good listener and could immediately recognise when someone was in pain or needed to talk. In a strange sort of way, Steve became our de facto counsellor. He knew what it was like to suffer and could relate to those who were troubled. Visitors would often spend as much time with Steve as with their relative/friend and many of them returned to the unit after the death of their relative, just to see Steve.

In the first few months of his stay Steve often asked to go home. Home to his friends at the boarding house who, incidentally, continued to visit right up to the time he died. I'm not sure whether Steve really did want to go home or whether he thought that going home would be a sign that things were getting better. We tried, but something always cropped up to stop the plan. If it wasn't pain or some other problem, it was the lack of a suitable room. Eventually, Steve stopped asking and I suspect it was because he knew he was not going to get better.

Steve was a great one for talking about his feats but never about himself, his family or his 'pain'. Then all of a sudden the floodgates opened and, not only did he talk, he insisted that it be recorded as he was sure it would bring him fame and fortune. He wanted someone to listen and record his story by hand rather than put it on tape and the reason soon became obvious. An elderly Irish Catholic volunteer (whom I will call Patricia) had befriended him and they had formed a wonderful relationship. She became a mother figure to him and he loved and respected her as he did his biological mother. Patricia came several days a week and recorded his sometimes horrific story verbatim. Her only proviso was that he refrain from the colourful language that invariably appeared as he became excited or agitated. When Patricia was not there others filled in, and I was one of the regular scribes. I could hardly believe some of the things he said but convinced myself that, if they were not fact, they were metaphors for his life and not lies.

After several weeks of non-stop talking, Steve started to withdraw and became overtly depressed. What started off as tales of bravado gradually changed to stories about home and family. Stirring up the past had brought more to the surface than he had bargained for. He began to have recurrent dreams of someone trying to slay him with a knife and these were so vivid and real that he was afraid to sleep at night. He used every ploy he knew to stay awake and it was not uncommon to see Steve in the smoking area at all hours of the night, smoking or eating or chatting to the night staff. He talked about his fear of dying and for the first time started to cry.

He wanted to see his parents who'd been in regular phone contact but had not yet visited. They lived interstate but now they began to visit regularly and this was the start of a healing process for Steve. I don't know what they talked about but it was clear their visits meant a lot to Steve. He started to glow but his body was wasting quickly. The tumour was quite massive and the pain was obviously bad, but the only time he complained was when the fear of dying overwhelmed him.

As the outer life fades the inner life becomes more intense.

VICTOR FRANKL

By now Steve held almost celebrity status within the palliative care unit. A party planned for his birthday had to be held in an adjoining building that had a room large enough to house the masses. Family, staff, patients and visitors joined in the celebration. Steve received more gifts on that one birthday than he'd had for the previous ten years. As he lay, confined to bed, surrounded by people, smiling his anything but Colgate smile, opening gifts, talking without swearing, I reminisced about that initial visit many months earlier. I wondered how many more people there were like Steve, who just need to feel loved and valued.

Steve's tumour had grown to such a size it was pressing on nerves and other painful structures. As a result he could neither lie flat nor sit upright. Only a few positions gave him brief periods of comfort. Despite this, he collared me one day and said he had not been to the beach for years and would like to see one before he got too sick. How sick do you have to get, was my immediate thought. But his enthusiasm was childlike so I spoke to the nurses, volunteers and ambulance officers and they all thought it was a great idea. They organised ambulance transport and an accompanying crew, made up of Patricia, one other volunteer and myself.

They made the long trip to Maroubra (20–30 kilometres) and I arranged to meet them there. Steve and his entourage duly arrived. His pale, gaunt face was painted with sunscreen and he wore an ill-fitting hat. The ambulance officer wheeled him onto the concourse and found a shady spot where Steve could look at the surf and the few board riders. It was a beautiful day but I had little time to soak up the scenery as Steve had me trotting to the local shops. He ate very little but insisted we savour the delights of Pluto Pups and Dim Sims.

Patricia sat by him except for a brief time when Steve released her so that she and the other volunteer could walk along the promenade. Steve enjoyed the outing but pain and discomfort limited his stay to just over an hour. He did not complain of pain but simply said he would like to go back to 'his bed'.

Steve had completed all that he needed to do. He was at peace with the world, his family and most of all he was at peace with himself. The layers of anger, bitterness, hatred and disregard had peeled away to reveal a vulnerable, frightened, compassionate human being, still with faults but faults he could now recognise and no longer needed to defend. As wasted as he was, it was another three months before Steve died. His funeral service was held in the same room as his birthday with just as many people present. But instead of laughter there were tears and instead of bearing gifts we gathered to acknowledge the gifts Steve had given us all. Steve had completed a journey I would have thought impossible—indeed, it may not have happened had he not had as much time as he did.

Lead us into darkness that we may find what lies concealed.

Michael Leunig, *The Prayer Tree*

What is unusual about Steve's story is the length of time he had to contemplate his life before he died. One year is a long time to be dying. Many people live longer with a life-threatening diagnosis but, unlike Steve, they often create distractions that temporarily relegate dying to the background. Steve had no distractions—no surgery or chemotherapy, no diets or complementary therapies and no one to search for miracle cures. Steve contemplated death in a way described by Leo Tolstoy in *The Death of Ivan Ilych*: 'Death drew his attention to itself, not in order to make him take some action but only that he should look at it, look at it straight in the face.' Steve did not want to look at death but it was always there, in the form of pain and paralysis, or in thoughts that he initially dared not confront. When these failed to draw his attention, death appeared through the medium of dreams and from these there was no escape. The dreams told Steve in no uncertain terms what he already knew, but had resisted.

Steve confronted his beasts and died a different person from the one who entered the unit twelve months earlier. 'People die the way they live', I have said. Steve may seem to contradict this but the fact is that people, including Steve, do not change because they are dying. We simply see another side of them, not something new but something newly revealed. The situation is analogous to Michelangelo's comment about the magnificent sculptures he created. Beauty, he said, is already present within the stone and all he did was to remove the excess. Dying removes the excess that accumulates through life and reveals only what is already there. This indisputable fact underpins much of the healing that is possible when someone is dying. As they come to know this part of themselves, free of the excesses, the invisible thread that held their life together becomes visible, often for the very first time. To discover there is a pattern to life, no matter how disconnected or dysfunctional that life may have been, is often the catalyst for healing, responsible for what is otherwise seen as change. Removing the excess may afford the dying person the first opportunity to understand who they really are. This form of self-discovery is not only liberating but often leads to acceptance and self-forgiveness, the basic requirements for unconditional love. Love for oneself is a prerequisite for 'dying well'.

 For what is it to die but to stand naked in the wind and to melt in the sun.

KAHLIL GIBRAN

As a palliative care physician, one of my greatest concerns is that people with life-threatening illnesses in the 21st century will not have enough time to contemplate their life and to heal whatever needs to be healed. The cure imperative has become so strong and the belief in medicine so great, society now believes that many of today's illnesses are curable and, for those that are not, life can be prolonged through the marvels of medical science.

Medicine has grown enormously in stature over the past twenty years, but we all still die; my concern is that medicine's plans for the future push death further and further into the background. In failing to recognise the inevitability of death, it turns a blind eye to human suffering and deludes itself into believing that death is without meaning. Death is unwelcome, particularly when it steals up on us, surprising us like some figure emerging from the dark. But it is never without meaning. What meaning does life have if death is meaningless?

There is an enormous body of knowledge and literature about death. Of the many messages that come through, none stands out more than the words of Scott Peck: 'When we shy away from death, the ever changing nature of things, we inevitably shy away from life.' This reinforces the strong, close relationship between life and death, a relationship that has always existed but is increasingly neglected or denied in a world that attempts to redefine life at the expense of death. There can be no life without death or death without life— together they complete the cycle of life. Not surprisingly, then, preparing for death teaches us about life and helps us to lead a more fulfilling life. Laying claim to the fact that we will all one day die is what makes life as valuable as any treasure, and death the treasure chest that contains it.

Dying is one of the most important times in a person's life. Preparing for it means leading a full and good life, as best we can. To reflect on this life as it draws to an end is what brings completion. To relive all that has been beautiful or painful, to talk about relationships that have been replenishing and those that need healing, to face our beasts, to speak of the people we love and to remember the wondrous things that have filled our life. The most peaceful people I have seen die were those who, like Steve, had time to do all these things. Their life cycle was complete and, to quote Goethe, 'like all things ripe, were ready to die'.

If we can accept death as part of life, not just as the end to life, living and dying become inseparable. Rather than a shadow that hovers over life, death becomes the light that illuminates life.

 O man go die before thou diest,
So that thou shalt not have to suffer when thou shalt die,
Such a death that thou wilst enter into light,
Not a death through which thou wilst enter into the grave.

RUMI 1207–73

Appendix

Palliative Care Australia
PO Box 24 Deakin West ACT 2600
Phone 02 6232 4433
Fax 02 6232 4434
Email pcainc@pallcare.org.au
Website www.pallcare.org.au

ACT Hospice Palliative Care Society
PO Box 88 Civic Square ACT 2608
Phone 02 6273 9606
Fax 02 6273 9590
Email acthpc@bigpond.com.au

Palliative Care Association of NSW
PO Box 572 Kings Cross NSW 1340
Phone 02 9334 1891
Fax 02 9326 9328
Email palliativecare@nswcc.org.au

Northern Territory Hospice and Palliative Care Association
PO Box 42255 Casuarina NT 0811
Phone 08 8927 4888
Fax 08 8927 4990
Email c/-uvstop@cancernt.org.au

Palliative Care Queensland
494 Boundary St Spring Hill Qld 4000
Phone 07 3832 3522
Fax 07 3832 4485
Email info@pallcareqld.com

Palliative Care Council of South Australia
202 Greenhill Road Eastwood SA 5063
Phone 08 8291 4237
Fax 08 8291 4122
Email pallcare@adelaide.on.net
Website www.pallcare.asn.au

Tasmanian Association for Hospice and Palliative Care
PO Box 517 North Hobart Tas 7002
Phone 03 6224 3808
Fax 03 6223 5042
Email hospicesouth@telstra.easymail.com.au

Palliative Care Victoria
2nd Floor 182 Victoria Pde East Melbourne Vic 3002
Phone 03 9662 9644
Fax 03 9662 9722
Email info@pallcarevic.asn.au
Website www.pallcarevic.asn.au

Palliative Care WA
46 Ventnor Ave West Perth WA 6005
Phone 08 9212 4330
Fax 08 9212 4330
Email pcwainc@palliativecarewa.asn.au
Website www.palliativecarewa.asn.au

Lifeline—telephone counselling service
Phone 13 11 14

NALAG (National Association for Loss and Grief)—
Advocacy body but also offers counselling and education
services where and when possible
PO Box 379 Dubbo NSW 2830
PO Box 214 Essendon Vic 3040
Phone 02 9976 2803 (NSW)

Phone 03 9331 3555 (Vic)
Email nalagvic@vicnet.net.au
Website vicnet.net.au/~nalgvic

Compassionate Friends—support service for
bereaved parents
Phone 02 9290 2355 (NSW)
Phone 02 6286 6134 (ACT)
Phone 03 9888 4944 (Vic)
Phone 03 6261 4250 (Tas)
Phone 07 3252 2920 (Qld)
Phone 08 8351 0344 (SA)
Phone 08 9486 8711 (WA)

Carers Resource Centre—provides a range of information,
resources and support to carers
Phone 1800 242 636

Funeral Director—national advisory service and directory of
funeral services
Phone 1800 086 000

Registry of Births, Deaths and Marriages
Phone 1300 655 236 (NSW)
Phone 02 6207 0460 (ACT)
Phone 1300 369 367 (Vic)
Phone 03 6233 3793 (Tas)
Phone 07 3247 9203 (Qld)
Phone 08 8204 9599 (SA)
Phone 08 9264 1555 (WA)
Phone 08 8999 6119 (NT)

Centrelink
Phone 13 23 00
Website www.centrelink.gov.au

Bibliography

Albom M *Tuesdays with Morrie*
Sydney: Hodder, 1998

Bailey LW and Yates J *The Near-Death Experience* New York:
Routledge, 1996

Barbato M Bispectral index
monitoring in unconscious
palliative care patients *Journal of
Palliative Care* 2001;17(2):
102–108

Barks C *The Essential Rumi* San
Francisco: HarperCollins, 1995

Barrett W *Death Bed Visions*
Wellingborough,
Northamptonshire: Aquarian
Press, 1986

Callahan D *Pursuing a Peaceful Death*
Hastings Centre Report, 1993;
23(4): 33–38

Clerk NW *A Grief Observed*
London: Faber & Faber, 1961

Cohen M *Australian Family Physician*
2001; 30(1): 17–19

Cole R *Mission of Love* Melbourne:
Lothian, 1999

Collett M *At Home with Dying—A
Zen Hospice Approach* Boston:
Shambhala, 1999

d'Apice M *Noon to Nightfall*
Burwood, Victoria: Collins Dove,
1989

Darling D *After Life* London: Fourth
Estate Ltd, 1995

Dass R *Death is not an Outrage*
Colorado: Sounds True
Recordings, 1992

Dass R and Gorman P *How Can I
Help?* New York: Borzoi, 1985

De Hennezel M *Intimate Death*
London: Warner Books, 1997

Dowrick S *Intimacy and Solitude*
Melbourne: Heinemann, 1991

Frankl V *Man's Search for Meaning*
Boston: Beacon Press, 1959

Fromm E *The Art of Loving* London:
Unwin Books, 1957

Gibran K *The Prophet* London:
Heinemann, 1979

Grof S *Books of the Dead* London:
Thames & Hudson, 1994

Grof S *The Cosmic Game*
Melbourne: Hill of Content,
1998

Hinton J *Dying* Middlesex: Penguin,
1967

Jones GC *Magnanimous Despair*
Mount Nebo, Qld: Boombana,
1998

Jouvet M *The Paradox of Sleep*
London: The MIT Press, 1999

Kazan A *Reflections on Dying* Sydney:
private publication, 1999

Kearney M *Mortally Wounded*
Dublin: Marino Books, 1996

Kellehear A *Death and Dying in
Australia* Melbourne: Oxford
University Press, 2000

Kellehear A *Eternity and Me*
Melbourne: Hill of Content,
2000

Kessler D *The Rights of the Dying*
New York: HarperCollins, 1997

Kübler-Ross E *On Death and Dying*
London: Tavistock Publications,
1970

Kübler-Ross E *To Live Until We Say Goodbye* London: Prentice Hall, 1978

Kübler-Ross E *On Children and Death* New York: Collier Books, 1983

Kübler-Ross E and Kessler D *Life Lessons* New York: Scribner, 2000

Lamerton R *Care of the Dying* Middlesex: Penguin, 1980

Lee EA *A Good Death* Old Noarlunga, South Australia: Stirling Press, 1996

Leunig M *Common Prayer Collection* North Blackburn, Victoria: Collins Dove, 1991

Levine S *Who Dies* New York: Doubleday, 1982

Levine S *Healing into Life and Death* New York: Doubleday, 1987

Lowentahl R *Cancer—What to do about it* Melbourne: Lothian, 1996

McKissock M and McKissock D *Coping with Grief* Sydney: ABC Books, 1985

May R *Man's Search for Himself* New York: Delta, 1973

May R *Freedom and Destiny* New York: WW Norton, 1981

Merikle PM and Daneman M Memory for unconsciously perceived events: evidence from anaesthetised patients. *Consciousness and Cognition* 1996; 5(4): 526–541

Mindell A *Coma—Key to Awakening* Boston: Shambhala, 1989

Moore T *Care of the Soul* New York: HarperCollins, 1992

Noll P *In the Face of Death* New York: Viking, 1989

O'Donohue J *Anam Cara* Sydney: Bantam, 1999

Osis K and Haraldsson E *At the Hour of Our Death* Norwalk, Connecticut: Hastings House, 1977

Reanney D *The Death of Forever* London: Souvenir Press, 1995

Remen RN *Kitchen Table Wisdom* Sydney: Pan Macmillan, 1996

Reoch R *Dying Well* Sydney: Hodder & Stoughton, 1997

Rinpoche S *The Tibetan Book of Living and Dying* Sydney: Random House, 1992

Sankar A *Dying at Home* London: The Johns Hopkins University Press, 1991

Stephenson JS *Death, Grief and Mourning* New York: Free Press, 1985

Sutherland C *Within the Light* Sydney: Bantam Books, 1993

Sutherland C *Children of the Light* Sydney: Bantam Books, 1995

Tarakson S *What to Do When Someone Dies* Marrickville NSW: Choice Books, 2001

Tobin DT *Peaceful Dying* New York: Perseus Books, 1999

Tolstoy L *The Death of Ivan Ilyich* London: Penguin Books, 1960

Wilber K *Grace and Grit* Melbourne: Collins Dove, 1991

Zukau G *The Seat of the Soul* London: Rider, 1990

Index